Virtual Clinical Excursions—General Hospital

for

deWit:
Medical-Surgical Nursing: Concepts and Practice, Second Edition

Virtual Clinical Excursions—General Hospital

for

deWit:
Medical-Surgical Nursing: Concepts and Practice,
Second Edition

Workbook prepared by

Kim D. Cooper, RN, MSN
Ivy Tech Community College
Terre Haute, Indiana

software developed by

Wolfsong Informatics, LLC
Tucson, Arizona

ELSEVIER
SAUNDERS

3251 Riverport Lane
Maryland Heights, Missouri 63043

VIRTUAL CLINICAL EXCURSIONS—GENERAL HOSPITAL FOR
DEWIT: MEDICAL-SURGICAL NURSING: CONCEPTS AND PRACTICE,
SECOND EDITION
Copyright © 2013, 2009 by Saunders, an imprint of Elsevier Inc.

ISBN: 978-1-4557-2616-5

Notice

ISBN: 978-1-4557-2616-5

Vice President eSolutions—Nursing: *Tom Wilhelm*
Director, Simulation Solutions: *Jeff Downing*
Associate Content Development Specialist: *Krissy Prysmiki*
Publishing Services Manager: *Jeff Patterson*
Senior Project Manager: *Tracey Schriefer*

Printed in the United States of America

Last digit is the print number: 9 8 7 6 5 4 3

Workbook
prepared by

Kim D. Cooper, RN, MSN
Ivy Tech Community College
Terre Haute, Indiana

Textbook

Susan C. deWit, MSN, RN, CNS, PHN
Formerly, Instructor of Nursing
El Centro College
Dallas, Texas

Table of Contents
Virtual Clinical Excursions Workbook

Getting Started

Lessons

Table of Contents
deWit:
Medical-Surgical Nursing: Concepts and Practice, 2nd Edition

Getting Started

GETTING SET UP WITH VCE ONLINE

The product you have purchased is part of the Evolve Learning System. Please read the following information thoroughly to get started.

■ HOW TO ACCESS YOUR VCE RESOURCES ON EVOLVE

There are two ways to access your VCE Resources on Evolve:

1. If your instructor has enrolled you into your VCE Evolve Resources you will receive an email with your registration details.

2. If your instructor has asked you to self-enroll into your VCE Evolve Resources they will provide you with your Course ID (for example: 1479_jdoe73_0001). You will then need to follow the instructions at https://evolve.elsevier.com/cs/studentEnroll.html.

There are two ways to access the virtual hospital portion of *Virtual Clinical Excursions:* online through the Evolve VCE Resources or via the CD-ROM that accompanies the VCE workbook. Instructions for both are provided below.

■ HOW TO ACCESS THE ONLINE VIRTUAL HOSPITAL

The online virtual hospital is available through the Evolve VCE Resources. There is no software to download or install: the online virtual hospital runs within your internet browser, using a popup window.

ONLINE: TECHNICAL REQUIREMENTS

- Broadband connection (DSL or cable)
- 1024 x 768 screen resolution
- Mozilla Firefox 18.0, Internet Explorer 9.0, Google Chrome and Safari 5 or higher
  Note: Pop-up blocking software/settings must be disabled.
- Adobe Acrobat Reader
- Additional technical requirements can be found at http://evolvesupport.elsevier.com.

■ HOW TO ACCESS THE VIRTUAL HOSPITAL VIA THE CD-ROM

The virtual hospital is available through the CD-ROM located in the back of your print workbook.

CD-ROM: MINIMUM SYSTEM REQUIREMENTS

WINDOWS®

Windows Vista®, XP, 2000 (Recommend Windows XP/2000)
Pentium® III processor (or equivalent) @ 600 MHz (Recommend 800 MHz or better)
256 MB of RAM (Recommend 1 GB or more for Windows Vista)
800 x 600 screen size (Recommend 1024 x 768)
Thousands of colors
12x CD-ROM drive

Note: Windows Vista and XP require administrator privileges for installation.

MACINTOSH® (*Note:* This CD will not work in Mac Lion 10.7)

MAC OS X (up to 10.6)
Apple Power PC G3 @ 500 MHz or better
128 MB of RAM (Recommend 256 MB or more)
800 x 600 screen size (Recommend 1024 x 768)
Thousands of colors
12x CD-ROM drive
Stereo speakers or headphones

CD-ROM: INSTALLATION INSTRUCTIONS

WINDOWS

1. Insert the *Virtual Clinical Excursions* CD-ROM.
2. The setup screen should appear automatically if the current product is not already installed. Windows Vista users may be asked to authorize additional security prompts.
3. Follow the onscreen instructions during the setup process.

    If the setup screen does *not* appear automatically (and *Virtual Clinical Excursions* has not been installed already):
    a. Click the **My Computer** icon on your desktop or on your Start menu.
    b. Double-click on your CD-ROM drive.
    c. If installation does not start at this point:
       (1) Click the **Start** icon on the taskbar and select the **Run** option.
       (2) Type d:\setup.exe (where "d:\" is your CD-ROM drive) and press **OK**.
       (3) Follow the onscreen instructions for installation.

MACINTOSH

1. Insert the *Virtual Clinical Excursions* CD in the CD-ROM drive. The disk icon will appear on your desktop.
2. Double-click on the disk icon.
3. Double-click on the MAC run file.

Note: Virtual Clinical Excursions for Macintosh does not have an installation setup and can only be run directly from the CD.

CD-ROM: HOW TO USE VIRTUAL CLINICAL EXCURSIONS

WINDOWS

1. Double-click on the *Virtual Clinical Excursions* icon located on your desktop.
2. Or navigate to the program via the Windows Start menu.

Note: If your computer uses Windows Vista, right-click on the desktop shortcut and choose **Properties**. In the Compatibility Mode, check the box for "Run as Administrator."

MACINTOSH

1. Insert the *Virtual Clinical Excursions* CD in the CD-ROM drive. The disk icon will appear on your desktop.
2. Double-click on the disk icon.
3. Double-click on the MAC run file.

■ HOW TO ACCESS THE WORKBOOK

There are two ways to access the workbook portion of *Virtual Clinical Excursions:*

1. Print workbook
2. An electronic version of the workbook is available within the VCE Evolve Resources.

■ TECHNICAL SUPPORT

Technical support for *Virtual Clinical Excursions* is available by visiting the Technical Support Center at http://evolvesupport.elsevier.com or by calling 1-800-222-9570 inside the United States and Canada.

Trademarks: Windows® and Macintosh® are registered trademarks.

A QUICK TOUR

Welcome to *Virtual Clinical Excursions—Medical-Surgical*, a virtual hospital setting in which you can work with multiple complex patient simulations and also learn to access and evaluate the information resources that are essential for high-quality patient care. The virtual hospital, Pacific View Regional Hospital, has realistic architecture and access to patient rooms, a Nurses' Station, and a Medication Room.

■ BEFORE YOU START

Make sure you have your textbook nearby when you use *Virtual Clinical Excursions*. You will want to consult topic areas in your textbook frequently while working with the virtual hospital and workbook.

■ HOW TO SIGN IN

- Enter your name on the Student Nurse identification badge.
- Now choose one of the four periods of care in which to work. In Periods of Care 1 through 3, you can actively engage in patient assessment, entry of data in the electronic patient record (EPR), and medication administration. Period of Care 4 presents the day in review. Highlight and click the appropriate period of care. (For this quick tour, choose **Period of Care 1: 0730-0815**.)
- This takes you to the Patient List screen (see the How to Select a Patient section below). Only the patients on the Medical-Surgical Floor are available. Note that the virtual time is provided in the box at the lower left corner of the screen (0730, since we chose Period of Care 1).

Note: If you choose to work during Period of Care 4: 1900-2000, the Patient List screen is skipped since you are not able to visit patients or administer medications during the shift. Instead, you are taken directly to the Nurses' Station, where the records of all the patients on the floor are available for your review.

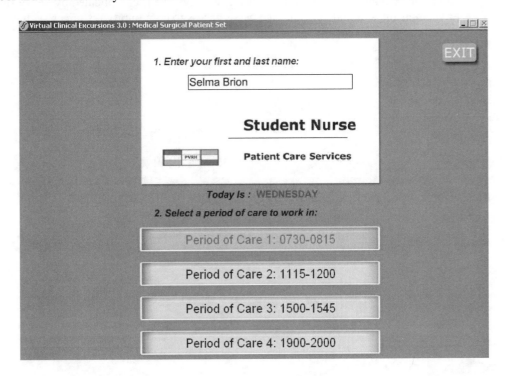

■ PATIENT LIST

MEDICAL-SURGICAL UNIT

Harry George (Room 401)
Osteomyelitis—A 54-year-old Caucasian male admitted from a homeless shelter with an infected leg. He has complications of type 2 diabetes mellitus, alcohol abuse, nicotine addiction, poor pain control, and complex psychosocial issues.

Jacquline Catanazaro (Room 402)
Asthma—A 45-year-old Caucasian female admitted with an acute asthma exacerbation and suspected pneumonia. She has complications of chronic schizophrenia, noncompliance with medication therapy, obesity, and herniated disc.

Piya Jordan (Room 403)
Bowel obstruction—A 68-year-old Asian female admitted with a colon mass and suspected adenocarcinoma. She undergoes a right hemicolectomy. This patient's complications include atrial fibrillation, hypokalemia, and symptoms of meperidine toxicity.

Clarence Hughes (Room 404)
Degenerative joint disease—A 73-year-old African-American male admitted for a left total knee replacement. His preparations for discharge are complicated by the development of a pulmonary embolus and the need for ongoing intravenous therapy.

Pablo Rodriguez (Room 405)
Metastatic lung carcinoma—A 71-year-old Hispanic male admitted with symptoms of dehydration and malnutrition. He has chronic pain secondary to multiple subcutaneous skin nodules and psychosocial concerns related to family issues with his approaching death.

Patricia Newman (Room 406)
Pneumonia—A 61-year-old Caucasian female admitted with worsening pulmonary function and an acute respiratory infection. Her chronic emphysema is complicated by heavy smoking, hypertension, and malnutrition. She needs access to community resources such as a smoking cessation program and meal assistance.

■ HOW TO SELECT A PATIENT

- You can choose one or more patients to work with from the Patient List by checking the box to the left of the patient name(s). For this quick tour, select Piya Jordan and Pablo Rodriguez. (In order to receive a scorecard for a patient, the patient must be selected before proceeding to the Nurses' Station.)
- Click on **Get Report** to the right of the medical records number (MRN) to view a summary of the patient's care during the 12-hour period before your arrival on the unit.
- After reviewing the report, click on **Go to Nurses' Station** in the right lower corner to begin your care. (*Note:* If you have been assigned to care for multiple patients, you can click on **Return to Patient List** to select and review the report for each additional patient before going to the Nurses' Station.)

Note: Even though the Patient List is initially skipped when you sign in to work for Period of Care 4, you can still access this screen if you wish to review the shift report for any of the patients. To do so, simply click on **Patient List** near the top left corner of the Nurses' Station (or click on the clipboard to the left of the Kardex). Then click on **Get Report** for the patient(s) whose care you are reviewing. This may be done during any period of care.

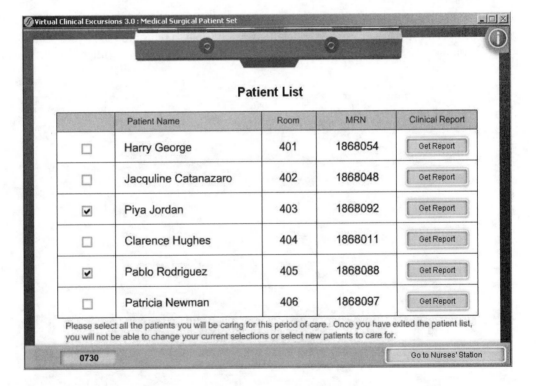

■ HOW TO FIND A PATIENT'S RECORDS

NURSES' STATION

Within the Nurses' Station, you will see:

1. A clipboard that contains the patient list for that floor.
2. A chart rack with patient charts labeled by room number, a notebook labeled Kardex, and a notebook labeled MAR (Medication Administration Record).
3. A desktop computer with access to the Electronic Patient Record (EPR).
4. A tool bar across the top of the screen that can also be used to access the Patient List, EPR, Chart, MAR, and Kardex. This tool bar is also accessible from each patient's room.
5. A Drug Guide containing information about the medications you are able to administer to your patients.
6. A Laboratory Guide containing normal value ranges for all laboratory tests you may come across in the virtual patient hospital.
7. A tool bar across the bottom of the screen that can be used to access the Floor Map, patient rooms, Medication Room, and Drug Guide.

As you run your cursor over an item, it will be highlighted. To select, simply click on the item. As you use these resources, you will always be able to return to the Nurses' Station by clicking on the **Return to Nurses' Station** bar located in the right lower corner of your screen.

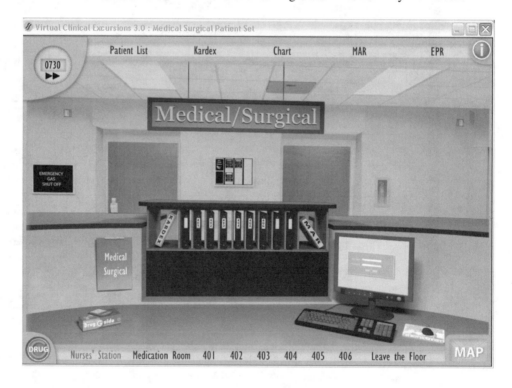

MEDICATION ADMINISTRATION RECORD (MAR)

The MAR icon located on the tool bar at the top of your screen accesses current 24-hour medications for each patient. Click on the icon and the MAR will open. (*Note:* You can also access the MAR by clicking on the MAR notebook on the far right side of the book rack in the center of the screen.) Within the MAR, tabs on the right side of the screen allow you to select patients by room number. Be careful to make sure you select the correct tab number for *your* patient rather than simply reading the first record that appears after the MAR opens. Each MAR sheet lists the following:

- Medications
- Route and dosage of each medication
- Times of administration of each medication

Note: The MAR changes each day. Expired MARs are stored in the patients' charts.

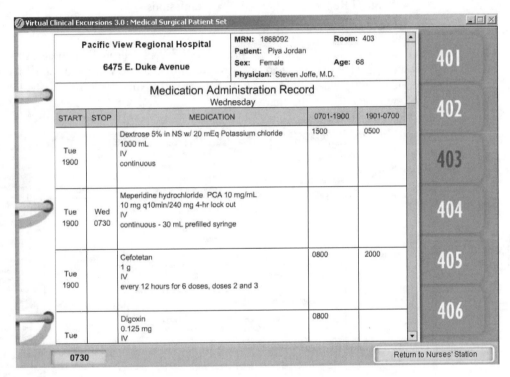

CHARTS

To access patient charts, either click on the **Chart** icon at the top of your screen or anywhere within the chart rack in the center of the Nurses' Station screen. When the close-up view appears, the individual charts are labeled by room number. To open a chart, click on the room number of the patient whose chart you wish to review. The patient's name and allergies will appear on the left side of the screen, along with a list of tabs on the right side of the screen, allowing you to view the following data:

- Allergies
- Physician's Orders
- Physician's Notes
- Nurse's Notes
- Laboratory Reports
- Diagnostic Reports
- Surgical Reports
- Consultations

- Patient Education
- History and Physical
- Nursing Admission
- Expired MARs
- Consents
- Mental Health
- Admissions
- Emergency Department

Information appears in real time. The entries are in reverse chronologic order, so use the down arrow at the right side of each chart page to scroll down to view previous entries. Flip from tab to tab to view multiple data fields or click on **Return to Nurses' Station** in the lower right corner of the screen to exit the chart.

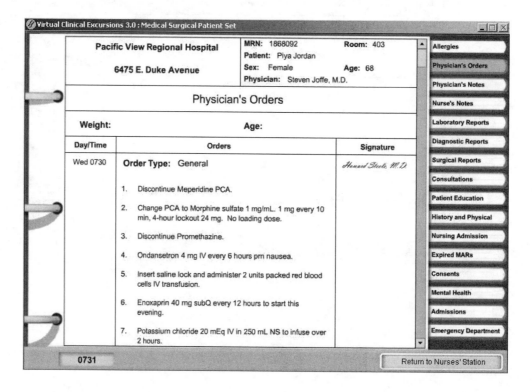

ELECTRONIC PATIENT RECORD (EPR)

The EPR can be accessed from the computer in the Nurses' Station or from the EPR icon located in the tool bar at the top of your screen. To access a patient's EPR:
- Click on either the computer screen or the **EPR** icon.
- Your username and password are automatically filled in.
- Click on **Login** to enter the EPR.
- *Note:* Like the MAR, the EPR is arranged numerically. Thus when you enter, you are initially shown the records of the patient in the lowest room number on the floor. To view the correct data for *your* patient, remember to select the correct room number, using the drop-down menu for the Patient field at the top left corner of the screen.

The EPR used in Pacific View Regional Hospital represents a composite of commercial versions being used in hospitals. You can access the EPR:
- to review existing data for a patient (by room number).
- to enter data you collect while working with a patient.

The EPR is updated daily, so no matter what day or part of a shift you are working, there will be a current EPR with the patient's data from the past days of the current hospital stay. This type of simulated EPR allows you to examine how data for different attributes have changed over time, as well as to examine data for all of a patient's attributes at a particular time. The EPR is fully functional (as it is in a real-life hospital). You can enter such data as blood pressure, breath sounds, and certain treatments. The EPR will not, however, allow you to enter data for a previous time period. Use the arrows at the bottom of the screen to move forward and backward in time.

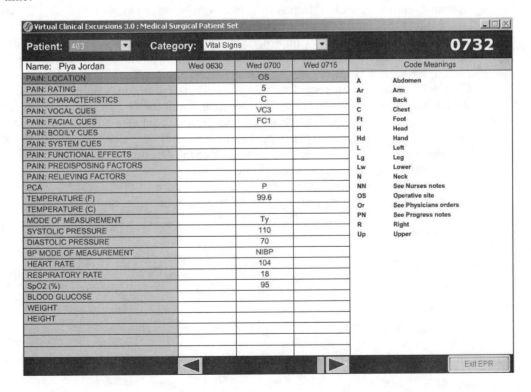

Name: Piya Jordan	Wed 0630	Wed 0700	Wed 0715	Code Meanings	
PAIN: LOCATION		OS		A	Abdomen
PAIN: RATING		5		Ar	Arm
PAIN: CHARACTERISTICS		C		B	Back
PAIN: VOCAL CUES		VC3		C	Chest
PAIN: FACIAL CUES		FC1		Ft	Foot
PAIN: BODILY CUES				H	Head
PAIN: SYSTEM CUES				Hd	Hand
PAIN: FUNCTIONAL EFFECTS				L	Left
PAIN: PREDISPOSING FACTORS				Lg	Leg
PAIN: RELIEVING FACTORS				Lw	Lower
PCA		P		N	Neck
TEMPERATURE (F)		99.6		NN	See Nurses notes
TEMPERATURE (C)				OS	Operative site
MODE OF MEASUREMENT		Ty		Or	See Physicians orders
SYSTOLIC PRESSURE		110		PN	See Progress notes
DIASTOLIC PRESSURE		70		R	Right
BP MODE OF MEASUREMENT		NIBP		Up	Upper
HEART RATE		104			
RESPIRATORY RATE		18			
SpO2 (%)		95			
BLOOD GLUCOSE					
WEIGHT					
HEIGHT					

At the top of the EPR screen, you can choose patients by their room numbers. In addition, you have access to 17 different categories of patient data. To change patients or data categories, click the down arrow to the right of the room number or category.

The categories of patient data in the EPR are as follows:

- Vital Signs
- Respiratory
- Cardiovascular
- Neurologic
- Gastrointestinal
- Excretory
- Musculoskeletal
- Integumentary
- Reproductive
- Psychosocial
- Wounds and Drains
- Activity
- Hygiene and Comfort
- Safety
- Nutrition
- IV
- Intake and Output

Remember, each hospital selects its own codes. The codes used in the EPR at Pacific View Regional Hospital may be different from ones you have seen in your clinical rotations. Take some time to acquaint yourself with the codes. Within the Vital Signs category, click on any item in the left column (e.g., Pain: Characteristics). In the far-right column, you will see a list of code meanings for the possible findings and/or descriptors for that assessment area.

You will use the codes to record the data you collect as you work with patients. Click on the box in the last time column to the right of any item and wait for the code meanings applicable to that entry to appear. Select the appropriate code to describe your assessment findings and type it in the box. (*Note:* If no cursor appears within the box, click on the box again until the blue shading disappears and the blinking cursor appears.) Once the data are typed in this box, they are entered into the patient's record for this period of care only.

To leave the EPR, click on **Exit EPR** in the bottom right corner of the screen.

■ VISITING A PATIENT

From the Nurses' Station, click on the room number of the patient you wish to visit (in the tool bar at the bottom of your screen). Once you are inside the room, you will see a still photo of your patient in the top left corner. To verify that this is the correct patient, click on the **Check Armband** icon to the right of the photo. The patient's identification data will appear. If you click on **Check Allergies** (the next icon to the right), a list of the patient's allergies (if any) will replace the photo.

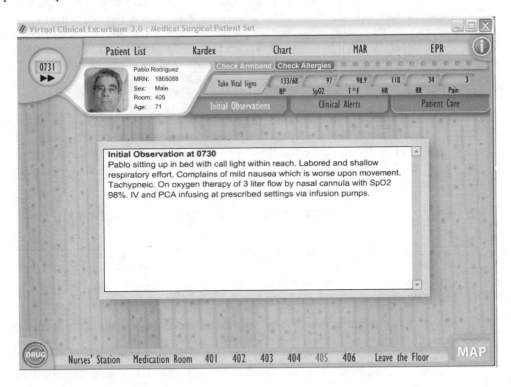

Also located in the patient's room are multiple icons you can use to assess the patient or the patient's medications. A virtual clock is provided in the upper left corner of the room to monitor your progress in real time. (*Note:* The fast-forward icon within the virtual clock will advance the time by 2-minute intervals when clicked.)

- The tool bar across the top of the screen allows you to check the **Patient List**, access the **EPR** to check or enter data, and view the patient's **Chart**, **MAR**, or **Kardex**.

- The **Take Vital Signs** icon allows you to measure the patient's up-to-the-minute blood pressure, oxygen saturation, temperature, heart rate, respiratory rate, and pain level.

- Each time you enter a patient's room, you are given an Initial Observation report to review (in the text box under the patient's photo). These notes are provided to give you a "look" at the patient as if you had just stepped into the room. You can also click on the **Initial Observations** icon to return to this box from other views within the patient's room. To the right of this icon is **Clinical Alerts**, a resource that allows you to make decisions about priority medication interventions based on emerging data collected in real time. Check this screen throughout your period of care to avoid missing critical information related to recently ordered or STAT medications.

- Clicking on **Patient Care** opens up three specific learning environments within the patient room: **Physical Assessment**, **Nurse-Client Interactions**, and **Medication Administration**.

- To perform a **Physical Assessment**, choose a body area (such as **Head & Neck**) from the column of yellow buttons. This activates a list of system subcategories for that body area (e.g., see **Sensory**, **Neurologic**, etc. in the green boxes). After you select the system you wish to evaluate, a brief description of the assessment findings will appear in a box to the right. A still photo provides a "snapshot" of how an assessment of this area might be done or what the finding might look like. For every body area, you can also click on **Equipment** on the right side of the screen.

- To the right of the Physical Assessment icon is **Nurse-Client Interactions**. Clicking on this icon will reveal the times and titles of any videos available for viewing. (*Note:* If the video you wish to see is not listed, this means you have not yet reached the correct virtual time to view that video. Check the virtual clock; you may return to access the video once its designated time has occurred—as long as you do so within the same period of care. Or you can click on the fast-forward icon within the virtual clock to advance the time by 2-minute intervals. You will then need to click again on **Patient Care** and **Nurse-Client Interactions** to refresh the screen.) To view a listed video, click on the white arrow to the right of the video title. Use the control buttons below the video to start, stop, pause, rewind, or fast-forward the action or to mute the sound.

- **Medication Administration** is the pathway that allows you to review and administer medications to a patient after you have prepared them in the Medication Room. This process is also addressed further in the *How to Prepare Medications* section below and in *Medications in the Detailed Tour.* For additional hands-on practice, see *Reducing Medication Errors* below the *Quick* and *Detailed Tours* in your resources.

■ HOW TO QUIT, CHANGE PATIENTS, OR CHANGE PERIODS OF CARE

How to Quit: From most screens, you may click the **Leave the Floor** icon on the bottom tool bar to the right of the patient room numbers. (*Note:* From some screens, you will first need to click an **Exit** button or **Return to Nurses' Station** before clicking **Leave the Floor**.) When the Floor Menu appears, click **Exit** to leave the program.

How to Change Patients or Periods of Care: To change patients, simply click on the new patient's room number. (You cannot receive a scorecard for a new patient, however, unless you have already selected that patient on the Patient List screen.) To change to a new period of care or to restart the virtual clock, click on **Leave the Floor** and then on **Restart the Program**.

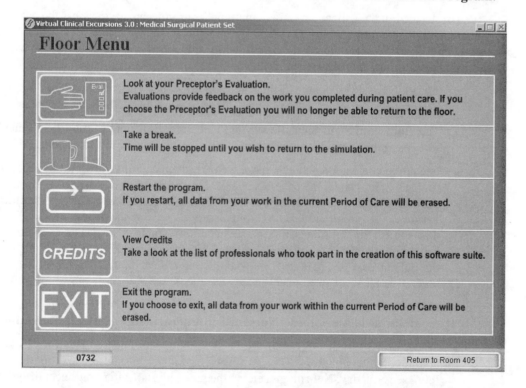

■ HOW TO PREPARE MEDICATIONS

From the Nurses' Station or the patient's room, you can access the Medication Room by clicking on the icon in the tool bar at the bottom of your screen to the left of the patient room numbers.

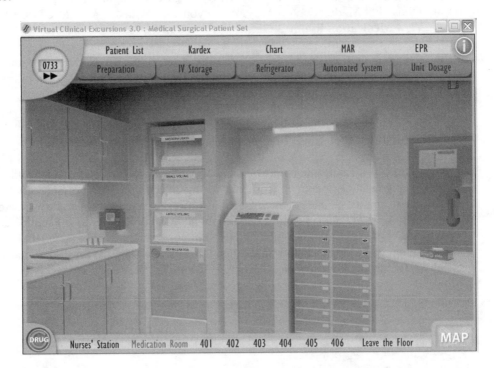

In the Medication Room you have access to the following (from left to right):

- A preparation area is located on the counter under the cabinets. To begin the medication preparation process, click on the tray on the counter or click on the **Preparation** icon at the top of the screen. The next screen leads you through a specific sequence (called the Preparation Wizard) to prepare medications one at a time for administration to a patient. However, no medication has been selected at this time. We will do this while working with a patient in *A Detailed Tour*. To exit this screen, click on **View Medication Room**.

- To the right of the cabinets (and above the refrigerator), IV storage bins are provided. Click on the bins themselves or on the **IV Storage** icon at the top of the screen. The bins are labeled **Microinfusion**, **Small Volume**, and **Large Volume**. Click on an individual bin to see a list of its contents. If you needed to prepare an IV medication at this time, you could click on the medication and its label would appear to the right under the patient's name. (*Note:* You can **Open** and **Close** any medication label by clicking the appropriate icon.) Next, you would click **Put Medication on Tray**. If you ever change your mind or decide that you have put the incorrect medication on the tray, you can reverse your actions by highlighting the medication on the tray and then clicking **Put Medication in Bin**. Click **Close Bin** in the right bottom corner to exit. **View Medication Room** brings you back to a full view of the entire room.

- A refrigerator is located under the IV storage bins to hold any medications that must be stored below room temperature. Click on the refrigerator door or on the **Refrigerator** icon at the top of the screen. Then click on the close-up view of the door to access the medications. When you are finished, click **Close Door** and then **View Medication Room**.

- To prepare controlled substances, click the **Automated System** icon at the top of the screen or click the computer monitor located to the right of the IV storage bins. A login screen will appear; your name and password are automatically filled in. Click **Login**. Select the patient for whom you wish to access medications; then select the correct medication drawer to open (they are stored alphabetically). Click **Open Drawer**, highlight the proper medication, and choose **Put Medication on Tray**. When you are finished, click **Close Drawer** and then **View Medication Room**.

- Next to the Automated System is a set of drawers identified by patient room number. To access these, click on the drawers or on the **Unit Dosage** icon at the top of the screen. This provides a close-up view of the drawers. To open a drawer, click on the room number of the patient you are working with. Next, click on the medication you would like to prepare for the patient, and a label will appear, listing the medication strength, units, and dosage per unit. To exit, click **Close Drawer**; then click **View Medication Room**.

At any time, you can learn about a medication you wish to prepare for a patient by clicking on the **Drug** icon in the bottom left corner of the medication room screen or by clicking the **Drug Guide** book on the counter to the right of the unit dosage drawers. The **Drug Guide** provides information about the medications commonly included in nursing drug handbooks. Nutritional supplements and maintenance intravenous fluid preparations are not included. Highlight a medication in the alphabetical list; relevant information about the drug will appear in the screen below. To exit, click **Return to Medication Room**.

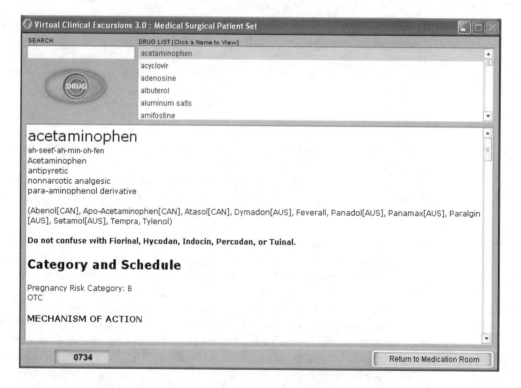

To access the MAR from the Medication Room and to review the medications ordered for a patient, click on the **MAR** icon located in the tool bar at the top of your screen and then click on the correct tab for your patient's room number. You may also click the **Review MAR** icon in the tool bar at the bottom of your screen from inside each medication storage area.

After you have chosen and prepared medications, go to the patient's room to administer them by clicking on the room number in the bottom tool bar. Inside the patient's room, click **Patient Care** and then **Medication Administration** and follow the proper administration sequence.

■ PRECEPTOR'S EVALUATIONS

When you have finished a session, click on **Leave the Floor** to go to the Floor Menu. At this point, you can click on the top icon (**Look at Your Preceptor's Evaluation**) to receive a score-card that provides feedback on the work you completed during patient care.

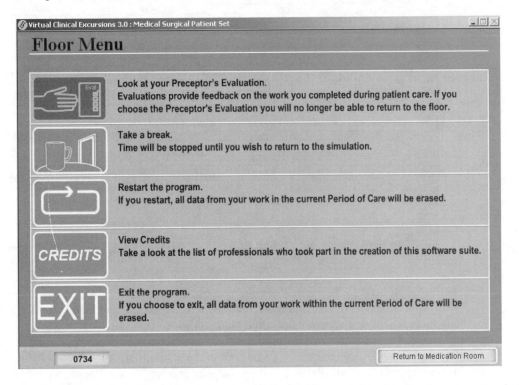

Evaluations are available for each patient you selected when you signed in for the current period of care. Click on the **Medication Scorecard** icon to see an example.

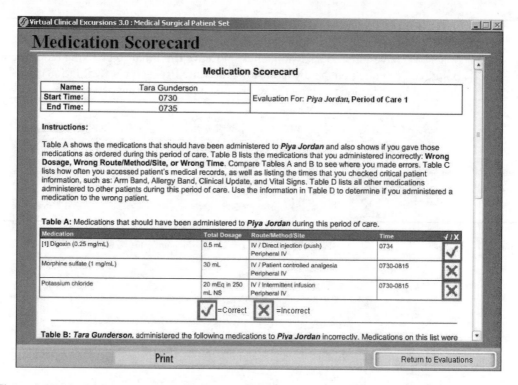

The scorecard compares the medications you administered to a patient during a period of care with what should have been administered. Table A lists the correct medications. Table B lists any medications that were administered incorrectly.

Remember, not every medication listed on the MAR should necessarily be given. For example, a patient might have an allergy to a drug that was ordered, or a medication might have been improperly transcribed to the MAR. Predetermined medication "errors" embedded within the program challenge you to exercise critical thinking skills and professional judgment when deciding to administer a medication, just as you would in a real hospital. Use all your available resources, such as the patient's chart and the MAR, to make your decision.

Table C lists the resources that were available to assist you in medication administration. It also documents whether and when you accessed these resources. For example, did you check the patient armband or perform a check of vital signs? If so, when?

You can click **Print** to get a copy of this report if needed. When you have finished reviewing the scorecard, click **Return to Evaluations** and then **Return to Menu**.

■ FLOOR MAP

To get a general sense of your location within the hospital, you can click on the **Map** icon found in the lower right corner of most of the screens in the *Virtual Clinical Excursions—Medical-Surgical* program. (*Note:* If you are following this quick tour step by step, you will need to **Restart the Program** from the Floor Menu, sign in again, and go to the Nurses' Station to access the map.) When you click the **Map** icon, a floor map appears, showing the layout of the floor you are currently on, as well as a directory of the patients and services on that floor. As you move your cursor over the directory list, the location of each room is highlighted on the map (and vice versa). The floor map can be accessed from the Nurses' Station, Medication Room, and each patient's room.

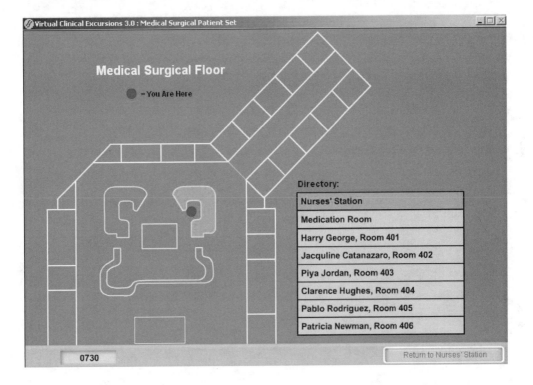

A DETAILED TOUR

If you wish to more thoroughly understand the capabilities of *Virtual Clinical Excursions—Medical-Surgical*, take a detailed tour by completing the following section. During this tour, we will work with a specific patient to introduce you to all the different components and learning opportunities available within the software.

■ WORKING WITH A PATIENT

Sign in for Period of Care 1 (0730-0815). From the Patient List, select Piya Jordan and Pablo Rodriguez; however, do not go to the Nurses' Station yet.

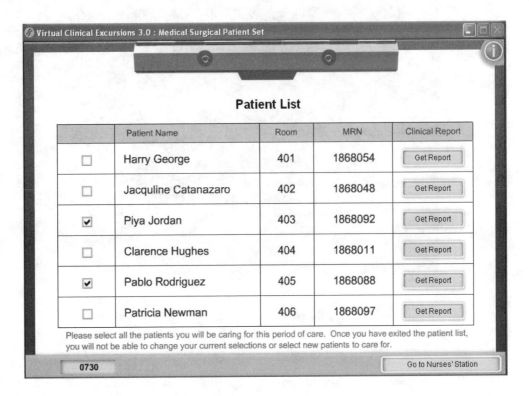

■ REPORT

In hospitals, when one shift ends and another begins, the outgoing nurse who attended a patient will give a verbal and sometimes a written summary of that patient's condition to the incoming nurse who will assume care for the patient. This summary is called a report and is an important source of data to provide an overview of a patient. Your first task is to get the clinical report on Piya Jordan. To do this, click **Get Report** in the far right column in this patient's row. From a brief review of this summary, identify the problems and areas of concern that you will need to address for this patient.

When you have finished noting any areas of concern, click **Go to Nurses' Station**.

■ CHARTS

You can access Piya Jordan's chart from the Nurses' Station or from the patient's room (403). From the Nurses' Station, click on the chart rack or on the **Chart** icon in the tool bar at the top of your screen. Next, click on the chart labeled **403** to open the medical record for Piya Jordan. Click on the **Emergency Department** tab to view a record of why this patient was admitted.

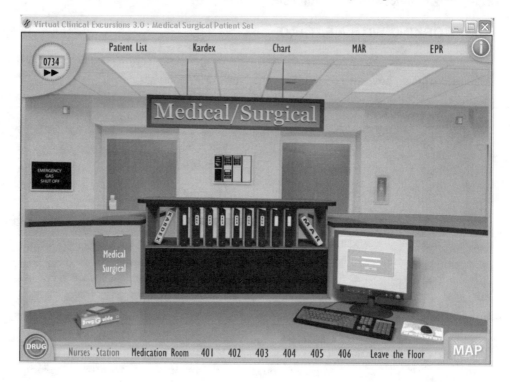

How many days has Piya Jordan been in the hospital?

What tests were done upon her arrival in the Emergency Department and why?

What was her reason for admission?

You should also click on **Diagnostic Reports** to learn what additional tests or procedures were performed and when. Finally, review the **Nursing Admission** and **History and Physical** to learn about the health history of this patient. When you are done reviewing the chart, click **Return to Nurses' Station**.

■ MEDICATIONS

Open the Medication Administration Record (MAR) by clicking on the **MAR** icon in the tool bar at the top of your screen. *Remember:* The MAR automatically opens to the first occupied room number on the floor—which is not necessarily your patient's room number! Since you need to access Piya Jordan's MAR, click on tab **403** (her room number). Always make sure you are giving the *Right Drug to the Right Patient!*

Examine the list of medications ordered for Piya Jordan. In the table below, list the medications that need to be given during this period of care (0730-0815). For each medication, note the dosage, route, and time to be given.

Time	Medication	Dosage	Route

Click on **Return to Nurses' Station**. Next, click on **403** on the bottom tool bar and then verify that you are indeed in Piya Jordan's room. Select **Clinical Alerts** (the icon to the right of Initial Observations) to check for any emerging data that might affect your medication administration priorities. Next, go to the patient's chart (click on the **Chart** icon; then click on **403**). When the chart opens, select the **Physician's Orders** tab.

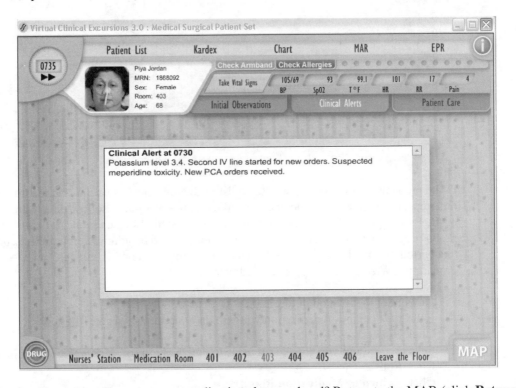

Review the orders. Have any new medications been ordered? Return to the MAR (click **Return to Room 403**; then click **MAR**). Verify that any new medications have been correctly transcribed to the MAR. Mistakes are sometimes made in the transcription process in the hospital setting, and it is sound practice to double-check any new order.

Are there any patient assessments you will need to perform before administering these medications? If so, return to Room 403 and click on **Patient Care** and then **Physical Assessment** to complete those assessments before proceeding.

Now click on the **Medication Room** icon in the tool bar at the bottom of your screen to locate and prepare the medications for Piya Jordan.

In the Medication Room, you must access the medications for Piya Jordan from the specific dispensing system in which each medication is stored. Locate each medication that needs to be given in this time period and click on **Put Medication on Tray** as appropriate. (*Hint:* Look in **Unit Dosage** drawer first.) When you are finished, click on **Close Drawer** and then on **View Medication Room**. Now click on the medication tray on the counter on the left side of the medication room screen to begin preparing the medications you have selected. (*Remember:* You can also click **Preparation** in the tool bar at the top of the screen.)

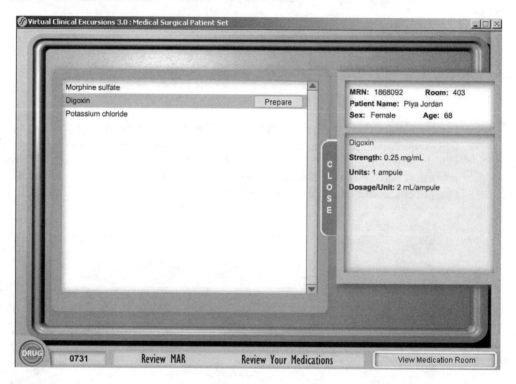

In the preparation area, you should see a list of the medications you put on the tray in the previous steps. Click on the first medication and then click **Prepare**. Follow the onscreen instructions of the Preparation Wizard, providing any data requested. As an example, let's follow the preparation process for digoxin, one of the medications due to be administered to Piya Jordan during this period of care. To begin, click to select **Digoxin**; then click **Prepare**. Now work through the Preparation Wizard sequence as detailed below:

> Amount of medication in the ampule: 2 mL.
> Enter the amount of medication you will draw up into a syringe: <u>0.5</u> mL.
> Click **Next**.
> Select the patient you wish to set aside the medication for: **Room 403, Piya Jordan**.
> Click **Finish**.
> Click **Return to Medication Room**.

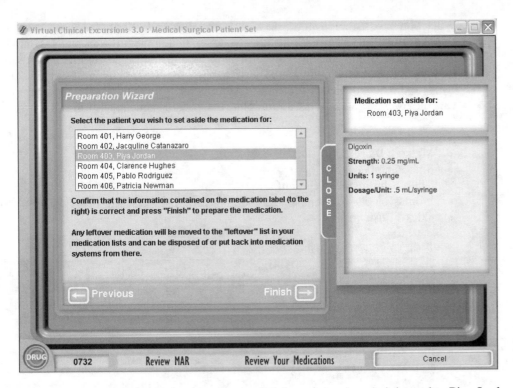

Follow this same basic process for the other medications due to be administered to Piya Jordan during this period of care. (*Hint:* Look in **IV Storage** and **Automated System**.)

PREPARATION WIZARD EXCEPTIONS

- Some medications in *Virtual Clinical Excursions—Medical-Surgical* are preprepared by the pharmacy (e.g., IV antibiotics) and taken to the patient room as a whole. This is common practice in most hospitals.
- Blood products are not administered by students through the *Virtual Clinical Excursions—Medical-Surgical* simulations since blood administration follows specific protocols not covered in this program.
- The *Virtual Clinical Excursions—Medical-Surgical* simulations do not allow for mixing more than one type of medication, such as regular and Lente insulins, in the same syringe. In the clinical setting, when multiple types of insulin are ordered for a patient, the regular insulin is drawn up first, followed by the longer-acting insulin. Insulin is always administered in a special unit-marked syringe.

Now return to Room 403 (click on **403** on the bottom tool bar) to administer Piya Jordan's medications.

At any time during the medication administration process, you can perform a further review of systems, take vital signs, check information contained within the chart, or verify patient identity and allergies. Inside Piya Jordan's room, click **Take Vital Signs**. (*Note:* These findings change over time to reflect the temporal changes you would find in a patient similar to Piya Jordan.)

When you have gathered all the data you need, click on **Patient Care** and then select **Medication Administration**. Any medications you prepared in the previous steps should be listed on the left side of your screen. Let's continue the administration process with the digoxin ordered for Piya Jordan. Click to highlight **Digoxin** in the list of medications. Next, click on the down arrow to the right of **Select** and choose **Administer** from the drop-down menu. This will activate the Administration Wizard. Complete the Wizard sequence as follows:

- Route: **IV**
- Method: **Direct Injection**
- Site: **Peripheral IV**
- Click **Administer to Patient** arrow.
- Would you like to document this administration in the MAR? **Yes**
- Click **Finish** arrow.

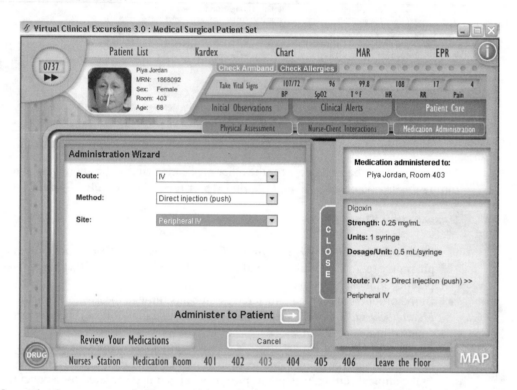

Your selections are recorded by a tracking system and evaluated on a Medication Scorecard stored under Preceptor's Evaluations. This scorecard can be viewed, printed, and given to your instructor. To access the Preceptor's Evaluations, click on **Leave the Floor**. When the Floor Menu appears, select **Look at Your Preceptor's Evaluation**. Then click on **Medication Scorecard** inside the box with Piya Jordan's name (see example on the following page).

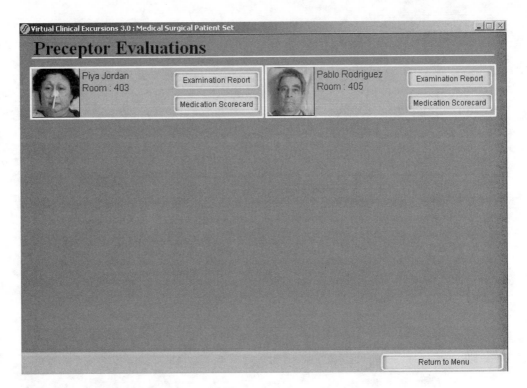

MEDICATION SCORECARD

- First, review Table A. Was digoxin given correctly? Did you give the other medications as ordered?
- Table B shows you which (if any) medications you gave incorrectly.
- Table C addresses the resources used for Piya Jordan. Did you access the patient's chart, MAR, EPR, or Kardex as needed to make safe medication administration decisions?
- Did you check the patient's armband to verify her identity? Did you check whether your patient had any known allergies to medications? Were vital signs taken?

When you have finished reviewing the scorecard, click **Return to Evaluations** and then **Return to Menu**.

■ **VITAL SIGNS**

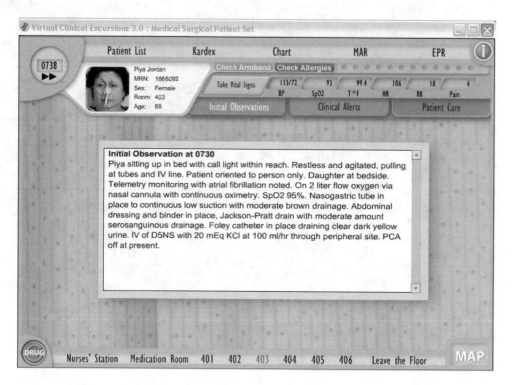

Vital signs, often considered the traditional "signs of life," include body temperature, heart rate, respiratory rate, blood pressure, oxygen saturation of the blood, and pain level.

Inside Piya Jordan's room, click **Take Vital Signs**. (*Note:* If you are following this detailed tour step by step, you will need to **Restart the Program** from the Floor Menu, sign in again for Period of Care 1, and navigate to Room 403.) Collect vital signs for this patient and record them below. Note the time at which you collected each of these data. (*Remember:* You can take vital signs at any time. The data change over time to reflect the temporal changes you would find in a patient similar to Piya Jordan.)

Vital Signs	Findings/Time
Blood pressure	
O$_2$ saturation	
Temperature	
Heart rate	
Respiratory rate	
Pain rating	

After you are done, click on the **EPR** icon located in the tool bar at the top of the screen. Your username and password are automatically provided. Click on **Login** to enter the EPR. To access Piya Jordan's records, click on the down arrow next to Patient and choose her room number, **403**. Select **Vital Signs** as the category. Next, in the empty time column on the far right, record the vital signs data you just collected in Piya Jordan's room. If you need help with this process, refer to the Electronic Patient Record (EPR) section of the Quick Tour. Now compare these findings with the data you collected earlier for this patient's vital signs. Use these earlier findings to establish a baseline for each of the vital signs.

    a.   Are any of the data you collected significantly different from the baseline for a particular vital sign?

       Circle One: Yes   No

    b.   If "Yes," which data are different?

■ PHYSICAL ASSESSMENT

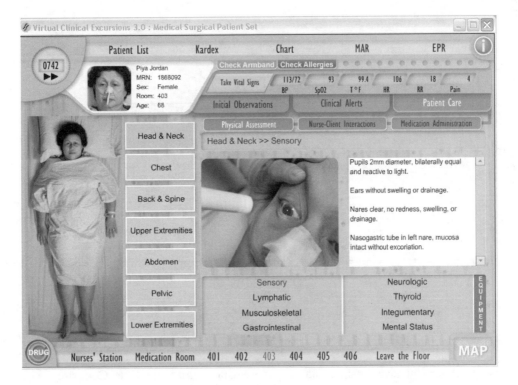

After you have finished examining the EPR for vital signs, click **Exit EPR** to return to Room 403. Click **Patient Care** and then **Physical Assessment**. Think about the information you received in the report at the beginning of this shift, as well as what you may have learned about this patient from the chart. Based on this, what area(s) of examination should you pay most attention to at this time? Is there any equipment you should be monitoring? Conduct a physical assessment of the body areas and systems that you consider priorities for Piya Jordan. For example, select **Head & Neck**; then click on and assess **Sensory** and **Lymphatic**. Complete any other assessment(s) you think are necessary at this time. In the following table, record the data you collected during this examination.

Area of Examination	Findings
Head & Neck Sensory	
Head & Neck Lymphatic	

After you have finished collecting these data, return to the EPR. Compare the data that were already in the record with those you just collected.

a. Are any of the data you collected significantly different from the baselines for this patient?

   Circle One: Yes   No

b. If "Yes," which data are different?

■ NURSE-CLIENT INTERACTIONS

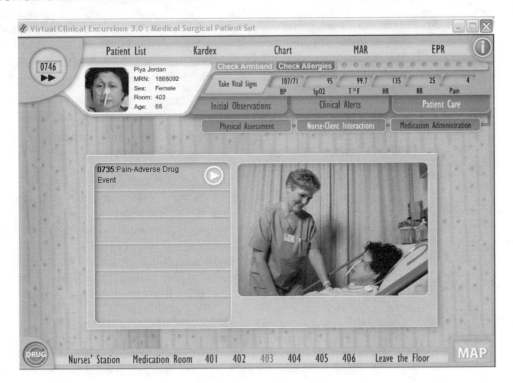

Click on **Patient Care** from inside Piya Jordan's room (403). Now click on **Nurse-Client Interactions** to access a short video titled **Pain—Adverse Drug Event**, which is available for viewing at or after 0735 (based on the virtual clock in the upper left corner of your screen; see *Note* below). To begin the video, click on the white arrow next to its title. You will observe a nurse communicating with Piya Jordan and her daughter. There are many variations of nursing practice, some exemplifying "best" practice and some not. Note whether the nurse in this interaction displays professional behavior and compassionate care. Are her words congruent with what is going on with the patient? Does this interaction "feel right" to you? If not, how would you handle this situation differently? Explain.

Note: If the video you wish to view is not listed, this means you have not yet reached the correct virtual time to view that video. Check the virtual clock; you may return to access the video once its designated time has occurred—as long as you do so within the same period of care. Or you can click on the fast-forward icon within the virtual clock to advance the time by 2-minute intervals. You will then need to click again on **Patient Care** and **Nurse-Client Interactions** to refresh the screen.

At least one Nurse-Client Interactions video is available during each period of care. Viewing these videos can help you learn more about what is occurring with a patient at a certain time and also prompt you to discern between nurse communications that are ideal and those that need improvement. Compassionate care and the ability to communicate clearly are essential components of delivering quality nursing care, and it is during your clinical time that you will begin to refine these skills.

■ COLLECTING AND EVALUATING DATA

Each of the activities you perform in the Patient Care environment generates a significant amount of assessment data. Remember that after you collect data, you can record your findings in the EPR. You can also review the EPR, patient's chart, videos, and MAR at any time. You will get plenty of practice collecting and then evaluating data in context of the patient's course.

Now, here's an important question for you:

> Did the previous sequence of exercises provide the most efficient way to assess Piya Jordan?

For example, you went to the patient's room to get vital signs, then back to the EPR to enter data and compare your findings with extant data. Next, you went back to the patient's room to do a physical examination, then again back to the EPR to enter and review data. If this back-and-forth process of data collection and recording seemed inefficient, remember the following:

- Plan all of your nursing activities to maximize efficiency, while at the same time optimizing the quality of patient care. (Think about what data you might need before performing certain tasks. For example, do you need to check a heart rate before administering a cardiac medication or check an IV site before starting an infusion?)

- You collect a tremendous amount of data when you work with a patient. Very few people can accurately remember all these data for more than a few minutes. Develop efficient assessment skills, and record data as soon as possible after collecting them.

- Assessment data are only the starting point for the nursing process.

Make a clear distinction between these first exercises and how you actually provide nursing care. These initial exercises were designed to involve you actively in the use of different software components. This workbook focuses on sensible practices for implementing the nursing process in ways that ensure the highest-quality care of patients.

Most important, remember that a human being changes through time, and that these changes include both the physical and psychosocial facets of a person as a living organism. Think about this for a moment. Some patients may change physically in a very short time (a patient with emerging myocardial infarction) or more slowly (a patient with a chronic illness). Patients' overall physical and psychosocial conditions may improve or deteriorate. They may have effective coping skills and familial support, or they may feel alone and full of despair. In fact, each individual is a complex mix of physical and psychosocial elements, and at least some of these elements usually change through time.

Thus it is crucial that you *DO NOT* think of the nursing process as a simple one-time, five-step procedure consisting of assessment, nursing diagnosis, planning, implementation, and evaluation. Rather, the nursing process should be utilized as a creative and systematic approach to delivering nursing care. Furthermore, because all living organisms are constantly changing, we must apply the nursing process over and over. Each time we follow the nursing process for an individual patient, we refine our understanding of that patient's physical and psychosocial conditions based on collection and analysis of many different types of data. *Virtual Clinical Excursions—Medical-Surgical* will help you develop both the creativity and the systematic approach needed to become a nurse who is equipped to deliver the highest-quality care to all patients.

REDUCING MEDICATION ERRORS

Earlier in the detailed tour, you learned the basic steps of medication preparation and administration. The following simulations will allow you to practice those skills further—with an increased emphasis on reducing medication errors by using the Medication Scorecard to evaluate your work.

Sign in to work at Pacific View Regional Hospital for Period of Care 1. (*Note:* If you are already working with another patient or during another period of care, click on **Leave the Floor** and then **Restart the Program**; then sign in.)

From the Patient List, select Clarence Hughes. Then click on **Go to Nurses' Station**. Complete the following steps to prepare and administer medications to Clarence Hughes.

- Click on **Medication Room** on the tool bar at the bottom of your screen.
- Click on **MAR** and then on tab **404** to determine medications that have been ordered for Clarence Hughes. (*Note:* You may click on **Review MAR** at any time to verify the correct medication order. Always remember to check the patient name on the MAR to make sure you have the correct patient's record. You must click on the correct room number tab within the MAR.) Click on **Return to Medication Room** after reviewing the correct MAR.
- Click on **Unit Dosage** (or on the Unit Dosage cabinet); from the close-up view, click on drawer **404**.
- Select the medications you would like to administer. After each selection, click **Put Medication on Tray**. When you are finished selecting medications, click **Close Drawer** and then **View Medication Room**.
- Click on **Automated System** (or on the Automated System unit itself). Click **Login**.
- On the next screen, specify the correct patient and drawer location.
- Select the medication you would like to administer and click on **Put Medication on Tray**. Repeat this process if you wish to administer other medications from the Automated System.
- When you are finished, click **Close Drawer** and **View Medication Room**.
- From the Medication Room, click on **Preparation** (or on the preparation tray).
- From the list of medications on your tray, highlight the correct medication to administer and click **Prepare**.
- This activates the Preparation Wizard. Supply any requested information; then click **Next**.
- Now select the correct patient to receive this medication and click **Finish**.
- Repeat the previous three steps until all medications that you want to administer are prepared.
- You can click on **Review Your Medications** and then on **Return to Medication Room** when ready. Once you are back in the Medication Room, go directly to Clarence Hughes' room by clicking on **404** at bottom of screen.
- Inside the patient's room, administer the medication, utilizing the six rights of medication administration. After you have collected the appropriate assessment data and are ready for administration, click **Patient Care** and then **Medication Administration**. Verify that the correct patient and medication(s) appear in the left-hand window. Highlight the first medication you wish to administer; then click the down arrow next to Select. From the drop-down menu, select **Administer** and complete the Administration Wizard by providing any information requested. When the Wizard stops asking for information, click **Administer to Patient**. Specify **Yes** when asked whether this administration should be recorded in the MAR. Finally, click **Finish**.

■ SELF-EVALUATION

Now let's see how you did during your medication administration!

- Click on **Leave the Floor** at the bottom of your screen. From the Floor Menu, select **Look at Your Preceptor's Evaluation**. Then click **Medication Scorecard**.

The following exercises will help you identify medication errors, investigate possible reasons for these errors, and reduce or prevent medication errors in the future.

1. Start by examining Table A. These are the medications you should have given to Clarence Hughes during this period of care. If each of the medications in Table A has a ✓ by it, then you made no errors. Congratulations!

If any medication has an X by it, then you made one or more medication errors.

Compare Tables A and B to determine which of the following types of errors you made: Wrong Dose, Wrong Route/Method/Site, or Wrong Time. Follow these steps:
   a. Find medications in Table A that were given incorrectly.
   b. Now see if those same medications are in Table B, which shows what you actually administered to Clarence Hughes.
   c. Comparing Tables A and B, match the Strength, Dose, Route/Method/Site, and Time for each medication you administered incorrectly.
   d. Then, using the form below, list the medications given incorrectly and mark the errors you made for each medication.

Medication	Strength	Dosage	Route	Method	Site	Time
	❑	❑	❑	❑	❑	❑
	❑	❑	❑	❑	❑	❑
	❑	❑	❑	❑	❑	❑
	❑	❑	❑	❑	❑	❑

2. To help you reduce future medication errors, consider the following list of possible reasons for errors.

- Did not check drug against MAR for correct medication, correct dose, correct patient, correct route, correct time, correct documentation.
- Did not check drug dose against MAR three times.
- Did not open the unit dose package in the patient's room.
- Did not correctly identify the patient using two identifiers.
- Did not administer the drug on time.
- Did not verify patient allergies.
- Did not check the patient's current condition or vital sign parameters.
- Did not consider why the patient would be receiving this drug.
- Did not question why the drug was in the patient's drawer.
- Did not check the physician's order and/or check with the pharmacist when there was a question about the drug or dose.
- Did not verify that no adverse effects had occurred from a previous dose.

Based on the list of possibilities you just reviewed, determine how you made each error and record the reason in the form below:

Medication	Reason for Error

3. Look again at Table B. Are there medications listed that are not in Table A? If so, you gave a medication to Clarence Hughes that he should not have received. Complete the following exercises to help you understand how such an error might have been made.

   a. Perhaps you gave a medication that was on Clarence Hughes' MAR for this period of care, without recognizing that a change had occurred in the patient's condition, which should have caused you to reconsider. Review patient records as necessary and complete the following form:

Medication	Possible Reasons Not to Give This Medication

   b. Another possibility is that you gave Clarence Hughes a medication that should have been given at a different time. Check his MAR and complete the form below to determine whether you made a Wrong Time error:

Medication	Given to Clarence Hughes at What Time	Should Have Been Given at What Time

c. Maybe you gave another patient's medication to Clarence Hughes. In this case, you made a Wrong Patient error. Check the MARs of other patients and use the form below to determine whether you made this type of error:

Medication	Given to Clarence Hughes	Should Have Been Given to

4. The Medication Scorecard provides some other interesting sources of information. For example, if there is a medication selected for Clarence Hughes but it was not given to him, there will be an X by that medication in Table A, but it will not appear in Table B. In that case, you might have given this medication to some other patient, which is another type of Wrong Patient error. To investigate further, look at Table D, which lists the medications you gave to other patients. See whether you can find any medications ordered for Clarence Hughes that were given to another patient by mistake. However, before you make any decisions, be sure to cross-check the MAR for other patients because the same medication may have been ordered for multiple patients. Use the following form to record your findings:

Medication	Should Have Been Given to Clarence Hughes	Given by Mistake to

5. Now take some time to review the medication exercises you just completed. Use the form below to create an overall analysis of what you have learned. Once again, record each of the medication errors you made, including the type of each error. Then, for each error you made, indicate specifically what you would do differently to prevent this type of error from occurring again.

Medication	Type of Error	Error Prevention Tactic

Submit this form to your instructor if required as a graded assignment, or simply use these exercises to improve your understanding of medication errors and how to reduce them.

Name: _____   Date: _____

KEY ICONS

The following icons are used throughout this workbook to help you quickly identify particular activities and assignments:

 Indicates a reading assignment—tells you which textbook chapter(s) you should read before starting each lesson

 Indicates a writing activity

 Marks the beginning of an interactive virtual hospital activity—signals you to return to your *Virtual Clinical Excursions* simulation

 Indicates additional virtual hospital activity instructions

 Indicates questions and activities that require you to consult your textbook

 Indicates the approximate time required to complete an exercise

LESSON 1

Fluids, Electrolytes, Acid-Base Balance, and Intravenous Therapy

Reading Assignment: Fluids, Electrolytes, Acid-Base Balance, and Intravenous Therapy (Chapter 3)

Patient: Patricia Newman, Medical-Surgical Floor, Room 406

Objectives:

1. Recall the various functions performed by body fluids.
2. Identify the body's mechanisms for fluid regulation.
3. Discuss three ways in which body fluids are continually being distributed among the fluid compartments.
4. Distinguish among the signs and symptoms of various electrolyte imbalances.
5. Discuss why older adults have more problems with fluid and electrolyte imbalances.
6. Discuss the steps in managing an intravenous infusion.
7. Identify isotonic intravenous fluids.
8. Discuss the principles of intravenous therapy.
9. Assess patients for signs of dehydration.
10. Apply your knowledge of normal laboratory values in order to recognize electrolyte imbalances.
11. Carry out interventions to correct an electrolyte imbalance.

Exercise 1

Writing Activity

30 minutes

1. Identify the average amounts of fluid lost by the body per day via the following routes.

   Urine: _____

   Perspiration: _____

   Feces: _____

   Expired air: _____

2. Match each of the following types of body fluids with its corresponding description.

Body Fluid Type	**Description**
_____ Extracellular fluid	a. Includes aqueous humor, saliva, and cerebrospinal fluid
_____ Intravascular fluid	b. Accounts for one-third of the total body fluid; transports water, nutrients, oxygen, and wastes
_____ Interstitial fluid	
_____ Transcellular fluid	c. Accounts for two-thirds of the total body fluid; the fluid contained within the cell walls
_____ Intracellular fluid	d. Fluid in the spaces surrounding the cells
	e. Fluid within the blood vessels; consists of plasma and fluid within blood cells

3. _____ Diffusion is a form of active transport. (True/False)

4. Which of the following are signs and symptoms associated with fluid volume deficit? Select all that apply.

   _____ Thirst

   _____ Thick saliva

   _____ Decreased hematocrit

   _____ Low urine specific gravity

   _____ Firm subcutaneous tissues

   _____ Postural hypotension

5. A patient experiencing nausea and vomiting is at greatest risk for developing which of the following acid-base imbalances?
   a. Metabolic acidosis
   b. Metabolic alkalosis
   c. Respiratory acidosis
   d. Respiratory alkalosis

6. The medications listed below are used to manage vomiting and diarrhea. Match each medication with its correct mode of action.

Medication	Mode of Action
_____ Diphenoxylate atropine (Lomotil)	a. Blocks receptors that act on the vomiting center
_____ Bismuth salts (Pepto-Bismol)	b. Depresses the central nervous system
_____ Loperamide HCl (Imodium)	c. Slows intestinal motility
_____ Prochlorperazine maleate (Compazine)	d. Decreases stool volume and increases stool bulk
_____ Hydroxyzine (Vistaril)	e. Inhibits prostaglandin synthesis responsible for gastrointestinal hypermotility

7. List the four general causes of edema.

8. A patient's serum calcium levels are elevated. Which of the following alterations in body system function may result?
   a. Alteration in blood coagulation
   b. Fluid retention
   c. Alteration in acid-base balance
   d. Reduced protein metabolism

9. If a patient has hyponatremia, which of the following clinical manifestations may result? Select all that apply.

_____ Fatigue

_____ Lethargy

_____ Decreased urine output

_____ Abdominal pain

_____ Increased urine pH

_____ Decreased blood pressure

10. The physician has prescribed a diet high in potassium. Which of the following foods will be the best source?
    a. Buttermilk
    b. Oranges
    c. Ham
    d. Tomato juice

11. _____ *Tonicity* is the term used to measure the concentration of vitamins in an intravenous solution. (True/False) (*Hint:* Refer to page 59 in your textbook.)

12. When monitoring the rate of flow for an intravenous infusion, the nurse must recognize factors that affect the infusion rate. Which of the following statements concerning intravenous infusions are correct? Select all that apply.

_____ Lowering the IV bag will increase the rate of flow.

_____ A full infusion bag will infuse more rapidly.

_____ Viscous fluids will flow more rapidly.

_____ The larger the diameter of the needle and tubing, the faster the flow.

13. Which of the following intravenous solutions provides the greatest number of calories?
    a. Dextrose in water 5%
    b. Dextrose in water 10%
    c. Dextrose in saline 5%
    d. Lactated Ringer's solution

14. _____ TIV dressings are changed at least every 72 hours. (True/False)

Exercise 2

Virtual Hospital Activity

45 minutes

- Sign in to work at Pacific View Regional Hospital on the Medical-Surgical Floor for Period of Care 2. (*Note:* If you are already in the virtual hospital from a pervious exercise, click on **Leave the Floor** and then on **Restart the Program** to get to the sign-in window.)
- From the Patient List, select Patricia Newman (Room 406).
- Click on **Get Report** and read the shift report.
- Click on **Go to Nurses' Station**.
- Click on **Chart** and then on **406**.
- Click on and review the **Nursing Admission**.

1. Why was Patricia Newman admitted to the hospital?

2. _____ The most accurate method of assessing Patricia Newman's level of hydration is to check for tenting. (True/False)

→ • Click on and review the **Laboratory Reports**.

3. Patricia Newman has a serum potassium level of _____.

4. What is the normal range for serum potassium level?
   a. 3.0-4.5 mEq/L
   b. 3.5-5.0 mEq/L
   c. 3.5-5.5 mEq/L
   d. 4.0-6.5 mEq/L

5. When discussing dietary intake with Patricia Newman, what foods can be suggested to increase her potassium levels? Select all that apply.

   _____ Dried fruits

   _____ Tomatoes

   _____ Winter squash

   _____ Spinach

   _____ Prune juice

   _____ Cheese

6. The correct term for a potassium level below 3.5 mEq/L is:
   a. hypocalcemia.
   b. hypercalcemia.
   c. hypokalemia.
   d. hyperkalemia.
   e. hyponatremia.
   f. hypernatremia.

7. Which of the following are roles of potassium in the body? Select all that apply. (*Hint:* See Table 3-3 in your textbook.)

   _____ Regulation of plasma acid-base balance

   _____ Maintenance of fluid osmolarity and volume within the cell

   _____ Transmission of nerve impulses

   _____ Synthesis and breakdown of glycogen

→ • Still in the Laboratory Reports section, review Patricia Newman's blood chemistry results.

8. Which of the following statements concerning the results of Patrician Newman's blood chemistry are correct? Select all that apply.

   _____ The sodium levels are moderately elevated.

   _____ The sodium levels are within normal limits.

   _____ The chloride levels are less than normal.

→ • Click on and review the **Physician's Orders**.

9. What intravenous fluids have been ordered by the physician?

10. The physician has ordered the intravenous solution to infuse at _____ mL/hr.

11. In a 24-hour period of time, Patricia Newman will receive _____ mL of intravenous fluids.
    a. 750
    b. 1000
    c. 1750
    d. 1800
    e. 2000

12. One liter of the prescribed intravenous fluids will provide Patricia Newman with approximately how many calories?
   a. 100
   b. 140
   c. 170
   d. 200

13. _____ The tonicity of the intravenous fluid prescribed for Patricia Newman is best described as hypertonic. (True/False)

➤ • Click on **Return to Nurses' Station**.
   • Click on **406** at the bottom of your screen; then click on **Check Armband**.

14. Patricia Newman is _____ years of age.

➤ • Review the Initial Observations at 1115.
   • Click on **Patient Care** and then on **Physical Assessment**.
   • Review the assessment of the patient's IV site by clicking on **Upper Extremities** and then on **Integumentary**.

15. Patricia Newman has a _____ IV in place.

16. Review Patricia Newman's condition. What are the primary rationales for the administration of intravenous fluids?

17. Which of the following manifestations at Patricia Newman's IV site would be consistent with infiltration? Select all that apply.

   _____ Warmth at IV site

   _____ Coolness at IV site

   _____ Edema surrounding site of insertion

   _____ Tenderness at IV site

18. _____ Patricia Newman's IV site demonstrates early signs of infiltration. (True/False)

➡ • Click on **Nurses' Station**.
- Click on **EPR** and then on **Login**.
- Select **406** from the Patient drop-down menu and **Intake and Output** from the Category drop-down menu.
- Review Patricia Newman's output.

19. What volume of urine must be produced in order to administer potassium?
    a. 10 mL/hour
    b. 30 mL/hour
    c. 50 mL/hour
    d. 75 mL/hour

20. _____ Patricia Newman's urinary output meets the required amount to administer potassium. (True/False)

21. _____ Patricia Newman's intravenous administration is infusing the prescribed amount. (True/False)

➡ • Click on **Exit EPR**.
- Click on **MAR** and then on tab **406** to review Patricia Newman's scheduled medications.

22. Identify the medication that will be administered by IV route.

23. The total volume of this medication infused with the IV in a 24-hour period will be:
    a. 25 mL.
    b. 50 mL.
    c. 75 mL.
    d. 100 mL.

24. The IV medication is premixed in a _____ solution.

Care of Surgical Patients: Preoperative and Intraoperative Care

⌒∞ **Reading Assignment:** Care of Preoperative and Intraoperative Surgical Patients
(Chapter 4)
Care of Postoperative Surgical Patients (Chapter 5)

Patient: Piya Jordan, Medical-Surgical Floor, Room 403

Objectives:

1. Identify the types of patients most at risk for surgical complications and state why each is at risk.
2. Explain the physical, emotional, and psychosocial preparation of patients for surgical procedures.
3. Plan and implement patient and family teaching to prevent postoperative complications.
4. Analyze the differences in the various types of anesthesia and list the advantages and disadvantages of each.
5. Describe the care of the patient in the preoperative, intraoperative, and postanesthesia phases of the surgical experience.

Exercise 1

Writing Activity

45 minutes

1. Match each of the following types of surgery with its correct purpose.

Type of Surgery	Purpose
_____ Diagnostic	a. To relieve symptoms of a disease process rather than to cure the disease
_____ Restorative	b. To determine the origin and cause of a disorder or the cell type for cancer
_____ Curative	
_____ Palliative	c. To alter or enhance personal appearance
_____ Cosmetic	d. To improve a patient's functional ability
	e. To resolve a health problem by repairing or removing the cause

2. The use of computerized, mechanical instruments is known as _____.

3. A patient is preparing to undergo a surgical procedure to repair a facial injury. Based on your knowledge, which of the following suffixes should be used to describe this type of procedure?
   a. -ectomy
   b. -lysis
   c. -plasty
   d. -pexy

4. Identify several patient variables that can affect surgical outcomes.

5. Identify topics that should be covered in a preoperative teaching session. (*Hint:* See pages 72-73 in your textbook.)

6. _____ The use of cell saver procedures would allow a Jehovah's Witness patient to undergo a major surgery and still uphold his or her religious beliefs. (True/False)

7. _____ Insulin is contraindicated in the preoperative phase. (True/False)

8. Patients planning to undergo surgery should discontinue taking herbal supplements _____

   to _____ weeks before surgery.

9. Assessing for the use of corticosteroid medications is vital in the care of the patient preparing for surgery. Which of the following implications can the use of corticosteroids have on the operative patient? Select all that apply.

   _____ Delay in wound healing

   _____ Alteration of fluid balance

   _____ Increase in blood clotting times

   _____ Reduction of respiratory secretions

   _____ Alteration of electrolyte balance

10. While preparing a patient for surgery, the nurse presents the surgical consent for the patient's signature. The patient reports that he does not understand what the physician told him about the rationale for the procedure. Which of the following responses/actions by the nurse is most appropriate?
    a. "This is just a formality. You can sign anyway."
    b. "Let me explain the procedure so that you can sign."
    c. "I will contact your physician so that you can ask for clarification."
    d. "You won't be able to get better without this surgery."

11. Which of the following patients are able to provide informed consent for surgery? Select all that apply.

    _____ A 101-year-old male

    _____ A married 17-year-old female

    _____ A 21-year-old female who has received preoperative medications

    _____ A 17-year-old male

    _____ A confused 34-year-old male

12. A patient is admitted to the clinical facility for an unexpected surgery. During the data collection, the nurse determines that the patient had toast and hot tea earlier in the day. How much fasting time is typically required before surgery after ingesting a meal of this type?
    a. 2 hours
    b. 4 hours
    c. 6 hours
    d. 8 hours

13. Prior to the surgery, _____ takes place to provide a period for final verification of vital information.

14. Which of the following are considered major functions of the circulating nurse during a surgical procedure? Select all that apply.

_____ Coordinates care, oversees the environment, and cares for the patient in the operating room

_____ Assists members of the surgical team with the ties on the backs of their gowns

_____ Monitors blood loss during surgery

_____ Maintains order and neatness on the instrument table

_____ Labels surgical instruments

_____ Prepares the patient's skin before draping

15. Which of the following are considered major functions of the scrub nurse during a surgical procedure? Select all that apply.

_____ Gathers all equipment for the procedure

_____ Obtains the surgical consent

_____ Provides preoperative education to the patient

_____ Gowns and gloves the surgeons upon entry into the operating room

_____ Monitors for breaks in the sterile technique

_____ Maintains the instrument table

16. During surgery, the atmosphere is cool. Which of the following statements best explains the rationale for this?
a. Keeping the room cool reduces the likelihood for the transmission of bacteria.
b. The cooled room promotes comfort for the surgical team members, who are wearing heavy surgical garments.
c. The cool temperature aids in reducing the body's metabolic rate.
d. Cooling the atmosphere reduces blood loss by the surgical patient.

17. During the surgical procedure, the circulating nurse monitors the patient for clinical manifestations of malignant hypothermia. Which of the following symptoms are consistent with the *early* onset of this phenomena? Select all that apply.

_____ Bradycardia

_____ Tachypnea

_____ Fever

_____ Flushed skin

_____ Chilling

Exercise 2

Virtual Hospital Activity

🕐 30 minutes

- Sign in to work at Pacific View Regional Hospital on the Medical-Surgical Floor for Period of Care 1. (*Note:* If you are already in the virtual hospital from a previous exercise, click on **Leave the Floor** and then on **Restart the Program** to get to the sign-in window.)
- From the Patient List, select Piya Jordan (Room 403).
- Click on **Get Report** and read the shift report.
- Click on **Go to Nurses' Station**.
- Click on **Chart** and then on **403**.
- Click on and review the **Nursing Admission**.

1. Why has Piya Jordan come to the hospital?

2. Piya Jordan's past medical history reflects disorders of which of the following body systems? Select all that apply.

_____ Pulmonary

_____ Cardiovascular

_____ Renal

_____ Neurologic

_____ Metabolic

_____ Integumentary

_____ Gastrointestinal

_____ Musculoskeletal

3. Piya Jordan is _____ years old.

→ • Click on and review the **Surgical Reports** and **Physician's Notes**.

4. What surgical procedure was performed on Piya Jordan?

5. Which of the following terms can be used to describe the type of surgical procedure performed on Piya Jordan? Select all that apply.

_____ Diagnostic

_____ Ablative

_____ Palliative

_____ Constructive

_____ Reconstructive

_____ Transplant

6. Which of the following best describes the urgency level of Piya Jordan's surgery?
   a. Elective
   b. Urgent
   c. Emergency

7. Piya Jordan received _____ anesthesia before surgery.

8. During the preoperative period, Piya Jordan was given midazolam as preoperative sedation. To which of the following categories does this medication belong? (*Hint:* Consult your nursing drug guide.)
   a. Opioid
   b. Anticonvulsant
   c. Nonbarbiturate
   d. Benzodiazepine

9. When these types of medications are administered, the nurse should monitor for what adverse reactions?

→ • Click on and review the **Laboratory Reports**.

10. Which of the following laboratory tests were performed on Piya Jordan during the preoperative phase? Select all that apply.

_____ Complete blood cell count (CBC)

_____ Urinalysis (UA)

_____ Serum cholesterol levels

_____ Type and crossmatch

_____ Arterial blood gases (ABG)

_____ Electrolyte panel

11. Laboratory testing completed during Piya Jordan's preoperative period reflected some abnormal values. Which of the following laboratory values were abnormal during the preoperative phase? Select all that apply.

_____ Red blood cell count (RBC)

_____ International normalized ratio (INR)

_____ Potassium

_____ Sodium

_____ Hemoglobin (Hgb)

_____ Hematocrit (Hct)

_____ Creatinine

_____ Prothrombin time (PT)

12. For which of the following complications is Piya Jordan at risk because of her INR reading?
    a. Urinary retention
    b. Pneumonia
    c. Paralytic ileus
    d. Hemorrhage

→ • Click on **Diagnostic Reports**.

13. Which of the following diagnostic tests were used to confirm the presence of Piya Jordan's abdominal mass? Select all that apply.

_____ Chest x-ray

_____ Kidney-ureter-bladder (KUB) scan

_____ Intravenous pyelogram (IVP)

_____ Colonoscopy

_____ Computed tomography (CT) scan of abdomen

→ • Click on **Surgical Reports**.

14. During the preoperative period, Piya Jordan received _____
as a prophylactic antibiotic.

15. _____ Piya Jordan has drug allergies that may influence the medications prescribed
by the physician in both the preoperative and postoperative phases.
(True/False)

→ • Click on **Physician's Orders**. Scroll to the notes for Tuesday at 0130.

16. Identify the intervention used to prepare Piya Jordan's bowel for the operative procedure.
a. Fleet (mineral oil) enema
b. No enema administered (because of the presence of the abdominal mass)
c. Soap suds enema
d. Oil retention enema

17. What type of catheter has the provider ordered preoperatively for Piya Jordan?

Exercise 3

Virtual Hospital Activity

15 minutes

• Sign in to work at Pacific View Regional Hospital on the Medical-Surgical Floor for Period
of Care 1. (*Note:* If you are already in the virtual hospital from a previous exercise, click on
Leave the Floor and then on **Restart the Program** to get to the sign-in window.)
• From the Patient List, select Piya Jordan (Room 403).
• Click on **Go to Nurses' Station**.
• Click on **403** at the bottom of the screen.
• Review the Initial Observations at 0730.
• Click on **Patient Care** and then on **Physical Assessment**.
• Complete a systems assessment for Piya Jordan by clicking on the body system categories
(yellow buttons) and subcategories (green buttons).

1. When performing the assessment on Piya Jordan's incision, the nurse should include which
of the following? Select all that apply.

_____ Approximation of the sutures

_____ Color of tissue surrounding the incision

_____ The presence of drainage from the incision

_____ Total number of sutures

_____ Odor of the incision

2. The recommended frequency for assessing Piya Jordan's vital signs (blood pressure, pulse, and respirations) during the postoperative period is:
   a. every 1 hour for 24 hours.
   b. every 4 hours for 48 hours.
   c. every shift for 48 hours.
   d. every 8 hours for 24 hours, then prn.

3. During the postoperative phase, Piya Jordan should be instructed/assisted to cough and

   deep-breathe every _____ hours.

→ • Click on **Chart** and then on **403**.
  • Click on and review the **Physician's Orders**.

4. _____ Piya Jordan's physician has ordered sequential compression devices for her legs. When the devices are removed for assessment and bathing, the nurse should massage her legs to promote circulation. (True/False)

5. Piya Jordan's surgeon ordered continued use of a nasogastric (NG) tube. Discuss the rationale for this.

6. The NG tube drainage should be assessed every _____ to _____ hours.

7. Piya Jordan has a Jackson-Pratt drain at her incision site. Which of the following statements about this device are correct? Select all that apply.

   _____ It was placed in Piya Jordan's incision while she was in the PACU.

   _____ It will reduce fluid accumulation between surfaces of the wound.

   _____ It is a small, pliable, flat latex tube used to promote drainage.

   _____ It is a closed drainage system.

   _____ It is an open drainage system.

   _____ It has a cartridge.

   _____ It has a bulb.

8. Identify several preventive interventions to reduce the occurrence of a wound infection.

Care of Patients with Pain

 Reading Assignment: Care of Patients with Pain (Chapter 7)

Patients: Harry George, Medical-Surgical Floor, Room 401
Pablo Rodriguez, Medical-Surgical Floor, Room 405

Objectives:

1. Demonstrate an understanding of the current view of pain as a specific entity requiring appropriate intervention.
2. Explain how pain perception is affected by personal situations and cultural backgrounds.
3. List the different pharmacologic approaches to pain management.
4. Analyze differences between acute and chronic pain and the management of each.

Exercise 1

 Writing Activity

🕐 30 minutes

1. _____ are pain receptors located in the skin, connective tissue, bones, joints, or muscles.

2. A _____ contains no medication (for example, sterile saline or sugar pills) and is very useful in assessing whether a patient actually has pain.

3. The _____ _____ is the point at which pain is perceived.

4. The length of time or the intensity of pain a person will endure before outwardly responding

   to it is known as _____ _____.

5. Place the phases of pain in the correct order of occurrence by matching the left and right columns below.

Phase	**Order of Occurrence**
_____ Perception	a. Phase 1
_____ Transduction	b. Phase 2
_____ Transmission	c. Phase 3
_____ Modulation	d. Phase 4

6. In managing pain, which of the following interventions is best implemented during the perception phase?
   a. Nonsteroidal antiinflammatory medications (NSAIDs)
   b. Opioids
   c. Drugs geared to blocking the neurotransmitter uptake
   d. Guided imagery

7. While caring for a patient experiencing chronic low-back pain, the nurse should understand that the physiologic structure of this pain is best described as:
   a. somatic.
   b. visceral.
   c. neuropathic.

8. _____ While caring for a patient who has recently been medicated for complaints of pain, it is appropriate for the nurse to ask the nursing assistant to recheck the patient's level of pain. (True/False)

9. A patient who has recently undergone surgery questions the use of narcotic analgesics and is concerned about becoming "hooked." Which of the following statements by the nurse is most therapeutic?
   a. "You should avoid the use of narcotics after the first postoperative day to reduce the incidence of addiction."
   b. "Addiction is an unfortunate but common event during the postoperative period."
   c. "Taking the ordered pain medicine every 6 hours will reduce the incidence of becoming addicted."
   d. "You should speak with your doctor about this concern."
   e. "Do you have a history of alcohol and drug dependence?"

10. Match each of the following characteristics with the type of pain it is most likely to be associated with.

Characteristic	Type of Pain
_____ Usually responds to commonly prescribed medical and nursing interventions	a. Acute pain
	b. Chronic pain
_____ May not be associated with an identified injury or event	
_____ Consists of discomfort lasting 1 to 2 months	
_____ Includes evidence of tissue damage	
_____ May not be reported	

11. List the types of tools available for assessing the presence and severity of pain.

12. When caring for the patient experiencing neuropathic pain, which of the following pharmacologic interventions are typically most successful? Select all that apply.

    _____ Opioids

    _____ Nonsteroidal antiinflammatory drugs (NSAIDs)

    _____ Tricyclic antidepressants

    _____ Corticosteroids

    _____ Anticonvulsants

13. When caring for the older patient, the nurse should be aware of which of the following factors associated with pain? Select all that apply.

    _____ Pain is a normal part of the aging process.

    _____ The older patient may believe that acknowledging pain is a sign of getting older.

    _____ Older patients may fear the cost of testing and treatment of a disorder.

    _____ Intramuscular injections are the best means of managing pain in the older population.

    _____ Older patients may report pain as "soreness" or "discomfort" rather than pain.

14. If the nurse is planning to use heat to manage a patient's pain, which of the following statements concerning the use of heat therapy is correct? Select all that apply.

_____ A warm compress should never be applied directly to the skin.

_____ Heat therapy is contraindicated in patients having peripheral vascular disease.

_____ Compresses and packs are usually left in place for 15 to 20 minutes.

_____ Heat applications may be moist or dry.

_____ Heat is a safe, effective means to manage pain related to a malignant tumor.

15. Cultural beliefs can affect a patient's perception of pain. However, remember that pain is individualized and perception and/or recognition of pain may not be characteristic of the patient's culture. Match each culture below with the characteristic response or belief relating to pain.

Culture	**Belief Relating to Pain**
_____ White (European; Caucasian)	a. May consider injections to manage pain too invasive of privacy
_____ Hispanic	b. Prefer to use nonnarcotic medications
_____ Black (African American, African native)	c. View pain as something to be controlled and expect prompt treatment
_____ Asian	d. Often feel pain is "God's will"
_____ American Indian (Native American)	e. May believe that laying-on of hands and prayer will help relieve pain
_____ Arab	f. Rely on traditional medicine men and the use of herbal preparations

Exercise 2

Virtual Hospital Activity

30 minutes

- Sign in to work at Pacific View Regional Hospital on the Medical-Surgical floor for period of Care 2. (*Note:* If you are already in the virtual hospital from a previous exercise, click on **Leave the Floor** and then on **Restart the Program** to get to the sign-in window.)
- From the Patient List, select Harry George (Room 401).
- Click on **Get Report** and read the shift report.
- Click on **Go to Nurses' Station** and then on **401**.
- Click on and review the **Clinical Alerts**.

1. When developing a plan of care for Harry George, which of the following nursing diagnoses is most appropriate and has the highest priority?
   a. Activity intolerance
   b. Ineffective role performance
   c. Ineffective coping
   d. Hopelessness
   e. Disturbed body image
   f. Acute pain

2. Harry George is reporting pain at a level of _____ on a _____-point scale.

3. The type of scale being used to assess Harry George's pain is known as a:
   a. visual analogue scale.
   b. numeric rating scale.
   c. verbal descriptor scale.
   d. linear pain continuum scale.

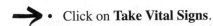 • Click on **Take Vital Signs**.

4. Discuss the relationship between Harry George's vital signs and his reports of pain.

 • Click on **Chart** and then on **401**.
- Click on and review the **Nursing Admission**, **History and Physical**, and **Physician's Notes**.

5. What are Harry George's medical diagnoses?

6. Which of the following terms does Harry George use to describe his discomfort at the time of admission? Select all that apply.

    _____ Intermittent

    _____ Continuous

    _____ Aching

    _____ Cramping

    _____ Throbbing

7. Based on the assessment data available, what type of pain is Harry George experiencing?
   a. Deep somatic pain
   b. Visceral pain
   c. Neuropathic pain

→ • Click on **Return to Room 401**.
   • Click on **MAR** and then on tab **401**.
   • Review Harry George's ordered medications.

8. Harry George was last medicated for pain at _____.

9. The route of administration for the pain medication was:
   a. oral (PO).
   b. intramuscular (IM).
   c. intravenous (IV).
   d. subcutaneous (subQ).

10. Harry George can be medicated for pain next at _____.

11. Which of the following medications is currently ordered by the physician to manage Harry George's pain?
   a. Oxycodone
   b. Hydromorphone hydrochloride
   c. Chlordiazepoxide hydrochloride
   d. Cefotaxime
   e. Thiamine

12. When the nurse is planning care for Harry George, how long after the administration of hydromorphone hydrochloride should interventions be performed to ensure maximum effectiveness of the drug? (*Hint:* Refer to the Drug Guide as necessary.)
   a. 15 minutes
   b. 15-30 minutes
   c. 30-60 minutes
   d. 2 hours
   e. 3 hours

13. Which method of administering analgesics will be most effective for Harry George: around the clock (ATC) or as needed (prn)? Why?

Exercise 3

 Virtual Hospital Activity

 30 minutes

- Sign in to work at Pacific View Regional Hospital for Period of Care 2. (*Note:* If you are already in the virtual hospital from a previous exercise, click on **Leave the Floor** and then on **Restart the Program** to get to the sign-in window.)
- From the Patient List, select Pablo Rodriguez (Room 405).
- Click on **Get Report** and read the shift report.
- Click on **Go to Nurses' Station** and then on **405**.
- Inside the patient's room, click on and review the **Clinical Alerts**.

1. Presently, Pablo Rodriguez is reporting a pain level of _____ on a 10-point scale.

 • Click on **Chart** and then on **405**.
- Click on and review the **Nursing Admission**, **Nurse's Notes**, **History and Physical**, and **Physician's Notes**.

2. What are Pablo Rodriguez's medical diagnoses?

 • Click on **Return to Room 405**.
- Click on **Patient Care** and then on **Physical Assessment**.
- Complete a head-to-toe physical assessment of Pablo Rodriguez by clicking on the body system categories (yellow buttons) and subcategories (green buttons).

3. Based on the assessment, which of the following are sources of discomfort for Pablo Rodriguez? Select all that apply.

_____ Condition of the oral cavity

_____ Constipation

_____ Ability to urinate

_____ Breathing

_____ Subcutaneous nodules

_____ Lymph nodes in the neck

→ • Click on **EPR** and then on **Login**.
  • Select **405** from the Patient drop-down menu and **Vital Signs** from the Category drop-down menu.
  • Review the information concerning Pablo Rodriguez's pain during this hospitalization.

4. During this hospitalization, the range of reported pain levels for Pablo Rodriguez has been

between _____ and _____.

5. Which of the following characteristics are used to describe Pablo Rodriguez's pain on Wednesday? Select all that apply.

_____ Ache

_____ Burning

_____ Constant

_____ Dull

_____ Electric

_____ Intermittent

_____ Internal

_____ Sharp

_____ Shooting

→ • Click on **Exit EPR**.
  • Now click on **MAR** and select tab **405**.
  • Review Pablo Rodriguez's ordered medications.

6. Listed below are medications ordered for Pablo Rodriguez. Match each medication with its correct classification. (*Hint:* Click on the **Drug Guide** icon or consult your nursing drug guide.)

Medication	**Classification**
_____ Morphine sulfate	a. Antiemetic
_____ Metoclopramide hydrochloride	b. Ammonia detoxicant
_____ Mineral oil	c. Schedule II narcotic analgesic
_____ Zolpidem	d. Laxative
_____ Dexamethasone	e. Schedule IV hypnotic
_____ Senna	f. Antiemetic
_____ Lactulose	g. Laxative-stimulant
_____ Ondansetron	h. Corticosteroid

7. What is the rationale for ordering two analgesics to manage Pablo Rodriguez's pain?
   a. Providing the IV push medication will reduce his dependence on the PCA pump.
   b. Having multiple analgesic orders will allow him to choose the medication he prefers.
   c. This is a standard order.
   d. Having two medications provides a means to manage breakthrough pain.

8. Opioids have been ordered to manage Pablo Rodriguez's pain. Which of the following best describes the manner in which these medications work?
   a. Opioids interfere with the relay of the pain signal across the synapse.
   b. Opioids inhibit prostaglandin synthesis.
   c. Opioids reduce serotonin availability to reduce pain occurrence.
   d. Opioids prevent and block the generation of the pain signals sent.

9. Identify the potential side effects associated with opioid use. Select all that apply.

   _____ Diarrhea

   _____ Constipation

   _____ Drowsiness

   _____ Nausea

   _____ Hypertension

   _____ Bradycardia

   _____ Diaphoresis

LESSON 4

Care of Patients with Cancer

 Reading Assignment: Care of Patients with Cancer (Chapter 8)

Patient: Pablo Rodriguez, Medical-Surgical Floor, Room 405

Objectives:

1. Identify characteristics of neoplastic growths.
2. Identify factors that may contribute to the development of a malignancy.
3. Identify practices that can promote prevention and early detection of cancer.
4. Describe the various treatment options for cancer.
5. Understand the stages of the grieving processes experienced by the dying patient.

Exercise 1

 Writing Activity

30 minutes

1. _____ According to the textbook, the incidence of lung cancer in men in the United States is declining. (True/False)

2. _____ The incidence of lung cancer in women is increasing. (True/False)

3. A _____ is the abnormal replication of cells that are not beneficial.

4. _____ refers to the moving of cancerous cells to other body sites.

5. Which of the following foods have been shown to reduce the risk for developing cancer? Select all that apply.

   _____ Broccoli

   _____ Carrots

   _____ Bananas

   _____ Grapefruit

   _____ Cabbage

   _____ Celery

6. A patient is concerned about his risk for the development of prostate cancer. Which of the following statements concerning this type of cancer is true?
   a. Patients with prostate cancer often report the incidence of nonspecific indigestion.
   b. It is associated with sun exposure.
   c. It becomes increasingly common after age 35.
   d. African-American men have a high incidence of this cancer.

7. Match each of the following malignant growth types with its correct description.

Malignant Growth	**Description**
_____ Sarcoma	a. Cancer of the blood-forming system
_____ Carcinoma	b. Arises from mesenchymal tissues (bone, muscles, and connective tissue)
_____ Leukemia	c. Originates in the epithelial tissues (skin and mucous membranes)
_____ Melanoma	
	d. Malignancy of the pigment cells of the skin

8. A patient asks at what age she should have her first mammogram. A review of the patient's history is devoid of any significant risk factors. According to the textbook, you should recommend to this patient that she have her first mammogram at:
   a. 25 years of age.
   b. 30 years of age.
   c. 40 years of age.
   d. 45 years of age.

9. Match each diagnostic test with its corresponding description. (*Hint:* Refer to pages 153-155 in your textbook.)

Diagnostic Test	Description
_____ Computed tomography (CT) scan	a. Noninvasive, high-frequency sound waves are used to examine external body structures.
_____ Radionuclide or isotope	b. A computer processes radiofrequency energy waves to assess spinal lesions, as well as cardiovascular and soft tissue abnormalities.
_____ Ultrasound testing	
_____ Magnetic resonance imaging (MRI)	c. Radiographs and computed scanning are used to provide images of structures at differing angles.
	d. A substance is injected; then the uptake is evaluated to identify areas of concern.

10. A 31-year-old woman who is sexually active and has no other risk factors asks how frequently she should have a Pap smear. A review of her medical history reveals normal Pap smears for the past 5 years. Based on this knowledge, which of the following time frames should be recommended in the nurse's response?
    a. Annually
    b. Every 2-3 years
    c. Every 3-5 years
    d. Every 6 months

11. List the seven warning signs of cancer.

12. If the physician has ordered the prostate-specific antigen (PSA) test, which of the following should be included in the information given to the patient? Select all that apply.

    _____ The patient will be NPO 8 hours before the test.

    _____ A clear liquid diet should be followed the day before the test.

    _____ The patient should have no sexual activity for 24 to 48 hours before the test.

    _____ A blood sample will be obtained before the digital examination.

    _____ A laxative will be prescribed and taken the evening before the test.

13. Before radiation therapy, the physician marked the skin of the patient. Which of the following instructions should be provided to the patient concerning these markings?
    a. "You may wash these marks with soap and water after this treatment."
    b. "Use a mild solution of rubbing alcohol and water to remove these marks."
    c. "Do not remove these marks."
    d. "Use lotion to soften the skin around these marks if needed."

14. The rate at which radiation therapies becomes less radioactive is termed

    _____-_____.

15. The complete blood cell profile of a patient diagnosed with cancer shows a reduction in the number of circulating platelets. Which of the following terms is used to describe this condition?
    a. Leukopenia
    b. Thrombocytopenia
    c. Anemia
    d. Neutropenia

16. A patient is experiencing diarrhea as a result of chemotherapy treatments. Which of the following best describes the underlying reason for this occurrence?
    a. The stomach contents dump rapidly into the colon.
    b. Absorption of nutrients is diminished by the gastrointestinal tract.
    c. The intestinal mucosa is inflamed.
    d. The lining of the stomach is beginning to atrophy.

Exercise 2

 Virtual Hospital Activity

 45 minutes

- Sign in to work at Pacific View Regional Hospital on the Medical-Surgical Floor for Period of Care 2. (*Note:* If you are already in the virtual hospital from a previous exercise, click on **Leave the Floor** and then on **Restart the Program** to get to the sign-in window.)
- From the Patient List, select Pablo Rodriguez (Room 405).
- Click on **Get Report** and read the shift report.
- Click on **Go to Nurses' Station**.
- Click on **405** at the bottom of your screen.
- Click on and review the **Clinical Alerts**.
- Click on **Chart** and then on **405**.
- Click on and review the **Nursing Admission**, **Physician's Orders**, and **History and Physical**.

1. What was Pablo Rodriguez's chief complaint at the time of admission?

2. What interventions were implemented to address these complaints?

3. What are Pablo Rodriguez's medical diagnoses?

4. How does Pablo Rodriguez report his prognosis?

5. _____ Pablo Rodriguez has a positive family history of cancer. (True/False)

6. Which of the following methods of treatment does Pablo Rodriguez report using to manage his cancer? Select all that apply.

_____ Surgery

_____ Radiation

_____ Chemotherapy

_____ Alternate therapies

_____ Complementary therapies

7. _____ is a means of cancer treatment that can be used to reduce or slow the growth of metastatic cells.

8. Which of the following best describes the mode of action/use of radiation therapy? Select all that apply.

_____ May be administered internally

_____ May be administered externally

_____ Used exclusively for palliative care

_____ Used to treat cancer that cannot be surgically removed

_____ Used to manage cancer that has spread to local lymph nodes

→ • Click on and review the **Physician's Orders** and **Physician's Notes**.

9. The physician has ordered a low-fat, bland diet. Discuss the implications of this ordered diet on Pablo Rodriguez's food preferences.

10. _____ Pablo Rodriguez's platelet levels are abnormal. (True/False)

11. _____ Pablo Rodriguez's white blood cell count (WBC) is reduced, reflecting immunosuppression. (True/False)

12. Which of the following complaints voiced by Pablo Rodriguez can be directly attributed to the results reflected in the complete blood cell count (CVC) results?
   a. Nausea
   b. Vomiting
   c. Constipation
   d. Fatigue

→ • Click on **Return to Room 405**.
   • Click on **Patient Care** and then on **Physical Assessment**.
   • Complete a head-to-toe assessment for Pablo Rodriguez by clicking on the body system categories (yellow buttons) and subcategories (green buttons).

13. At the time of his admission, Pablo Rodriguez reported being unable to tolerate oral intake. Which assessment findings support this report?

→ • Click on **Chart** and then on **405**.
  • Click on **Physician's Orders** and review the orders from Wednesday morning at 1100.

14. The physician ordered ondansetron hydrochloride for Pablo Rodriguez. Which of the following side effects associated with this medication may further complicate problems Pablo Rodriguez is currently facing? Select all that apply.

_____ Fatigue

_____ Excitability

_____ Diarrhea

_____ Urinary retention

_____ Constipation

_____ Blurred vision

15. What additional medication has been ordered to manage Pablo Rodriguez's nausea?

16. In addition to opioids, what medications may be used in the management of cancer pain?

Care of Patients with Disorders of the Respiratory System: Part 1

Reading Assignment: The Respiratory System (Chapter 13)
Care of Patients with Disorders of the Upper Respiratory
System (Chapter 14)
Care of Patients with Disorders of the Lower Respiratory
System (Chapter 15)

Patient: Patricia Newman, Medical-Surgical Floor, Room 406

Objectives:

1. Describe the various sounds that may be heard when auscultating the lung fields.
2. Review care of the patient with pneumonia.
3. Recognize abnormal blood chemistry values when providing care for the patient diagnosed with pneumonia.

Exercise 1

Writing Activity

15 minutes

1. The _____ _____ is an airtight compartment that encloses each lung.

2. The alveoli secrete a substance known as _____, which acts to reduce surface tension in the alveolar walls and promotes expansion with inspiration.

3. List several characteristics of individuals who are at a high risk for the development of a respiratory infection.

4. Describe several changes associated with aging that may increase the potential for complications in the older patient.

5. Which of the following tests may be used to assess the integrity of mechanical function and gas exchange function of the lungs?
   a. Pulmonary function tests
   b. Pulmonary angiography
   c. Computed tomography
   d. Mediastinoscopy

6. Match each of the following breath sounds with its correct description.

Breath Sound	Description
_____ Wheezes	a. Grating, scratching sounds, similar to a squeaky door
_____ Rhonchi	b. Whistling, musical, high-pitched sounds produced by air being forced through narrowed airways
_____ Crackles	
_____ Stridor	c. Coarse, low-pitched, sonorous, rattling sounds caused by secretions in larger air passages
_____ Pleural friction rub	d. Croaking sounds heard with partial obstruction in the upper air passages
	e. Sounds similar to rubbing hairs between fingers close to the ears

7. While performing a pulmonary assessment, the nurse identifies bronchovesicular breath sounds. Which of the following findings concerning these sounds are correct? Select all that apply.

_____ Low to moderate pitch

_____ Moderate to high pitch

_____ Presents with a soft, whooshing quality

_____ Inspiration two to three times the length of expiration

_____ Inspiration and expiration equal

_____ Loud, harsh, tubular quality

8. An abnormal respiratory sound is described as _____.

9. After the administration of an analgesic, which of the following types of respiratory patterns would be most anticipated?
   a. Biot's
   b. Kussmaul's
   c. Cheyne-Stokes
   d. Tachypnea
   e. Bradypnea

Exercise 2

Virtual Hospital Activity

45 minutes

- Sign in to work at Pacific View Regional Hospital on the Medical-Surgical Floor for Period of Care 3. (*Note:* If you are already in the virtual hospital from a previous exercise, click on **Leave the Floor** and on **Restart the Program** to get to the sign-in window.)
- From the Patient List, select Patricia Newman (Room 406).
- Click on **Get Report** and read the shift report.
- Click on **Go to Nurses' Station**.
- Click on **Chart** and then on **406**.
- Click on and review the **History and Physical**.

1. Why has Patricia Newman been admitted to the hospital?

2. What medical diagnoses are listed for Patricia Newman? (*Hint:* See the Impression section.)

3. Potential infectious causes of pneumonia include _____,

   _____, and _____.

4. The most common cause of bacterial pneumonia is _____.

5. Which of the following conditions and/or aspects of Patricia Newman's medical history have placed her at an increased risk for the development of pneumonia? Select all that apply.

   _____ Smoking

   _____ Hypertension

   _____ Osteoporosis

   _____ Social isolation

   _____ Hysterectomy

   _____ Emphysema

6. How much fluid intake should be included in Patricia Newman's care plan?
   a. Limited to reduce fluid retention.
   b. 1000-1200 mL per day
   c. 1500-2000 mL per day
   d. 2500-3000 mL per day

→ • Click on and review the **Laboratory Reports**.

7. Which of the following components of Patricia Newman's hematology test is abnormal?
   a. White blood cell count (WBC)
   b. Red blood cell count (RBC)
   c. Hemoglobin (Hgb)
   d. Hematocrit (Hct)
   e. Mean corpuscular volume (MCV)
   f. Platelets

8. Assess the values from the arterial blood gases (ABGs) drawn on Wednesday at 0600. Which of these values are abnormal? Select all that apply.

_____ PaO_2

_____ O_2 saturation

_____ $PaCO_2$

_____ pH

9. What is the identified cause of Patricia Newman's pneumonia?

→ • Click on **Return to Nurses' Station**.
  • Click on **406** at the bottom of your screen; review the Initial Observations at 1500.
  • Click on **Take Vital Signs** and review the findings.

10. Record Patricia Newman's vital signs below. (*Note:* Vital signs will vary depending on exact time they are taken.)

Temperature:

Heart rate:

Blood pressure:

Respiratory rate:

→ • Click on **Patient Care** and then on **Physical Assessment**.
  • Complete a systems assessment for Patricia Newman by clicking on the body system categories (yellow buttons) and subcategories (green buttons).

11. Identify findings on the systems assessment consistent with the diagnosis of pneumonia.

12. List several nursing interventions that may be implemented to improve airway clearance.

13. Cefotan has been ordered to treat Patricia Newman's pneumonia. Which of the following is a frequent side effect associated with this medication? (*Hint:* Refer to the Drug Guide.)
    a. Oral candidiasis
    b. Nausea
    c. Vomiting
    d. Rash
    e. Pruritus
    f. Thrombophlebitis

14. Which of the following occurrences will signal successful action by the ordered Cefotan? Select all that apply.

    _____ Increased red blood cell count

    _____ Decreased red blood cell count

    _____ Decreased temperature

    _____ Decreased O_2 saturation

    _____ Decreased blood pressure

    _____ Decreased white blood cell count

Care of Patients with Disorders of the Respiratory System: Part 2

Reading Assignment: The Respiratory System (Chapter 13)

Care of Patients with Disorders of the Upper Respiratory System (Chapter 14)

Care of Patients with Disorders of the Lower Respiratory System (Chapter 15)

Patient: Jacquline Catanazaro, Medical-Surgical Floor, Room 402

Objectives:

1. Describe the clinical manifestations associated with common respiratory disorders.
2. Review diagnostic tests and/or assessments that may be performed on a patient experiencing a respiratory disorder.
3. Discuss care of a patient with asthma.

Exercise 1

Writing Activity

 15 minutes

1. Match each of the following respiratory disorders with its appropriate description.

Respiratory Disorder	Description
_____ Atelectasis	a. Inflammation of the lung with consolidation and exudation
_____ Pleural effusion	b. Accumulation of fluid in the pleural space
_____ Hemothorax	c. A collapsed or incomplete expansion of alveoli
_____ Pneumothorax	d. An infectious, inflammatory, reportable disease that is chronic and commonly affects the lungs, although it may occur in other areas of the body
_____ Pneumonia	
_____ Asthma	e. An inflammatory response that constricts the bronchi, causing edema and increased sputum
_____ Emphysema	f. Bleeding into the pleural space secondary to chest trauma
_____ Tuberculosis	g. Pathologic accumulation of air in tissues or organs
	h. Air from the lung leaking into the pleural space or chest

2. _____ For the patient with asthma, an absence of wheezing during a period of respiratory distress is a positive sign. (True/False)

3. When managing the care of a patient suspected of having asthma, which of the following tests may be ordered to confirm a diagnosis? Select all that apply.

_____ Complete blood count (CBC)

_____ Serum electrolyte levels

_____ Arterial blood gas (ABG)

_____ Pulmonary function tests

_____ Chest radiograph

4. The pulse oximeter records a reading of the:
   a. level of the blood's hematocrit level.
   b. oxygen saturation of hemoglobin in the blood.
   c. body's level of $PaCO_2$.
   d. body's acid-base balance.

5. A patient has been scheduled to undergo a bronchoscopy. Which of the following statements concerning the procedure is correct?
   a. It is used to assess for sensitivity to iodine.
   b. An ice collar may be used for up to 48 hours postprocedure.
   c. The patient may feel a warm flush during the dye injection.
   d. The patient must be status nothing by mouth (NPO) at least 6 hours before the test.

6. The patient with chronic obstructive pulmonary disease (COPD) who does not have fluid

   restrictions should drink _____ to _____ glasses of noncaffeinated fluids per day.

Exercise 2

Virtual Hospital Activity

45 minutes

- Sign in to work at Pacific View Regional Hospital on the Medical-Surgical Floor for Period of Care 1. (*Note:* If you are already in the virtual hospital from a previous exercise, click on **Leave the Floor** and then on **Restart the Program** to get to the sign-in window.)
- From the Patient List, select Jacquline Catanazaro (Room 402).
- Click on **Get Report** and read the shift report.
- Click on **Go to Nurses' Station**.
- Click on **Chart**; then on **402**.
- Click on and review the **Nursing Admission** and **History and Physical**.

1. What are Jacquline Catanazaro's medical diagnoses?

2. Which of the following risk factors for the development of respiratory illnesses does Jacquline Catanazaro have? Select all that apply.

_____ Age

_____ History of travel

_____ Occupational exposures

_____ Smoking

_____ Family history

_____ Chronic respiratory disorder

3. Which of the following best describes Jacquline Catanazaro's type of asthma? (*Hint:* See pages 306 and 308 in your textbook.)
   a. Mild intermittent
   b. Mild persistent
   c. Moderate persistent
   d. Severe persistent

→ • Click on and review the **Diagnostic Reports** and **Laboratory Reports**.

4. Jacquline Catanazaro had arterial blood gases drawn on Tuesday at 0730. Which of the following charter results are abnormal? Select all that apply.

_____ PaO_2

_____ O_2 saturation

_____ $PaCO_2$

_____ pH

→ • Click on **Return to Nurses' Station**; then on **402** at the bottom of your screen.
   • Click on and review the **Initial Observations**.
   • Click on and review the **Clinical Alerts**.
   • Click on **Take Vital Signs** and review the findings.

5. What are Jacquline Catanazaro's current vital signs? (*Note:* Findings may vary depending on the exact time vital signs are taken.)

Temperature:

Heart rate:

Respiratory rate:

Blood pressure:

6. What is Jacquline Catanazaro's pulse oximeter reading?

→ • Click on **Patient Care** and then on **Physical Assessment**.
   • Complete a systems assessment by clicking on the body system categories (yellow buttons) and subcategories (green buttons).

7. Identify any abnormalities found during Jacquline Catanazaro's respiratory assessment.

8. Which of the following terms would best describe the "crackles" heard in Jacquline Catanazaro's lung fields?
   a. Continuous, sonorous sounds
   b. High-pitched, musical tones
   c. Low-pitched, whistling sounds
   d. Hairs being rubbed between fingers

9. Jacquline Catanazaro's respiratory assessment reflects the presence of wheezes. Which of the following best describes the underlying cause of the wheezing sound?
   a. Pulmonary hypoventilation
   b. Mucus in the bronchioles
   c. Inflammation of the pleura
   d. Bronchoconstriction
   e. Fluid overload

10. Jacquline Catanazaro is demonstrating an increased respiratory rate. Which of the following can result in an increased respiratory rate? Select all that apply.

   _____ Exercise

   _____ Fever

   _____ Alkalosis

   _____ Hypoxemia

   _____ Hypercapnia

11. Jacquline Catanazaro's skin is noted as being moist and clammy. What significance does this have in relation to her respiratory status?

12. Jacquline Catanazaro's condition is consistent with the late phase of an asthmatic attack. Which of the following factors are consistent with this phase? Select all that apply.

_____ Airway inflammation is reduced.

_____ Airway inflammation is pronounced.

_____ Red blood cells have infiltrated swollen tissues.

_____ This phase typically lasts only a few hours.

_____ The patient is at a heightened risk for an acute asthmatic attack.

13. Jacquline Catanazaro is demonstrating extreme agitation and anxiety. What is the impact of these behaviors on her condition?

➡ • Click on **Patient Care** and then on **Nurse-Client Interactions**.
   • Select and view the video titled **0730: Intervention—Airway**. (*Note:* Check the virtual clock to see whether enough time has elapsed. You can use the fast-forward feature to advance the time by 2-minute intervals if the video is not yet available. Then click again on **Patient Care** and on **Nurse-Client Interactions** to refresh the screen.)

14. Jacquline Catanazaro is experiencing an acute asthma attack. What has been planned to manage the onset?

15. Albuterol has been ordered to manage Jacquline Catanazaro's respiratory distress. When should she begin to feel relief from signs and symptoms? (*Hint:* Consult the Drug Guide.)
    a. Within 5-15 minutes
    b. Within 15-30 minutes
    c. Within 30-45 minutes
    d. Within 45-60 minutes

→ • Click on **Chart** and then on **402**.
   • Click on the **Physician's Orders** tab and review the orders for Monday at 1600.
   • Click on **Return to Room 402** and then click on the **Drug** icon in the lower right corner.
   • Review the information for the drugs that have been ordered for Jacquline Catanazaro.

16. What are the doses and routes of administration for each of the medications ordered to manage Jacquline Catanazaro's respiratory condition?

   Beclomethasone:

   Albuterol:

   Ipratropium bromide:

17. Match each of the prescribed medications with its correct mode of action.

Medication	**Mode of Action**
_____ Beclomethasone	a. Relief of bronchospasms
_____ Albuterol	b. Reduction of bronchial inflammation
_____ Ipratropium bromide	c. Control of secretions

18. When providing patient education concerning the use of beclomethasone, the nurse should tell the patient that which of the following side effects may occur?
   a. Throat irritation
   b. Productive cough
   c. Increased pulmonary secretions
   d. Skin rash
   e. Activity intolerance

19. When preparing Jacquline Catanazaro for discharge to home, which of the following guidelines should be included in the education provided? Select all that apply.

   _____ Following prescribed drug therapy

   _____ Limiting water intake to reduce pulmonary edema

   _____ Promptly reporting infections to physicians

   _____ Suspending activity if symptoms occur during exercise

   _____ Reviewing potential allergens in the home environment

Care of Patients with Cardiovascular Disorders

 Reading Assignment: The Cardiovascular System (Chapter 18)

Care of Patients with Hypertension and
Peripheral Vascular Disease (Chapter 19)

Care of Patients with Cardiac Disorders (Chapter 20)

Care of Patients with Coronary Artery Disease and
Cardiac Surgery (Chapter 21)

Patients: Piya Jordan, Medical-Surgical Floor, Room 403

Patricia Newman, Medical-Surgical Floor, Room 406

Objectives:

1. Describe the normal anatomy and physiology of the cardiovascular system.

2. Discuss the risk factors and incidence of cardiovascular disease.

3. Describe the diagnostic tests, specific techniques, and procedures for assessing the cardiovascular system.

4. Describe the pathophysiology, potential complications, and management of hypertension.

Exercise 1

 Writing Activity

🕐 45 minutes

1. _____ Heart disease is the number one killer of women. (True/False)

2. Which of the following recommendations are made to prevent cardiovascular disease in women? Select all that apply.

_____ Exercise at least 30 minutes 2 to 3 times per week.

_____ Maintain a body mass index (BMI) less than 25.

_____ Maintain high-density lipoproteins (HDL) levels less than 50 mg/dL.

_____ Maintain low-density lipoproteins (LDL) levels less than 129 mg/dL.

_____ Reduce the amounts of trans fats in the diet.

3. Which of the following risk factors for the development of cardiovascular disease are considered modifiable? Select all that apply.

_____ Heredity

_____ Gender

_____ Elevated cholesterol levels

_____ Excessive stress

_____ Diabetes

4. The point of maximal impulse is located between the:
   a. 3rd and 4th ribs.
   b. 4th and 5th ribs.
   c. 5th and 6th ribs.
   d. 6th and 7th ribs.

5. The _____ _____ is called the "pacemaker" of the heart.

6. _____ The patient with a pacemaker should be advised to take his or her pulse for 30 seconds daily during a period of exercise to ensure the pacemaker is functioning. (True/False)

7. A patient with a new pacemaker is concerned about the life of the battery in the device. What information should be given to the patient?
   a. Battery life is variable.
   b. The battery has an expected life span of 10 years.
   c. The battery is able to recharge continuously and will not wear out.
   d. The battery can be expected to last 6 to 9 years.

8. Which of the following measurements determine cardiac output? Select all that apply.

_____ Heart rate

_____ Respiratory rate

_____ Metabolic rate

_____ Amount of venous return

_____ Pressure in the arterial system

9. _____ Retained sodium causes a reduction in cardiac output. (True/False)

10. When a patient has a reduction in blood volume, the kidneys will secrete which of the following?
    a. Angiotensin
    b. Aldosterone
    c. Potassium
    d. Renin
    e. Creatinine

11. _____ An increase in blood viscosity will cause an increase in blood pressure.
    (True/False)

12. Match each of the following diagnostic tests with its correct description.

Diagnostic Test	Description
_____ Echocardiography	a. Small electrodes placed on the chest and extremities; records electrical impulses of the heart to determine rate, rhythm of heart, site of pacemaker, and presence of injury at rest
_____ Electrocardiography	
_____ Coronary angiography	b. A flexible catheter with a transducer in the tip is inserted into a coronary artery; determines patency of coronary arteries and presence of collateral circulation
_____ Coronary ultrasound	
_____ Venogram	c. Metal wand that emits sonar waves is guided over the chest while the patient is supine; useful in evaluating size, shape, and position of structures and movement within the heart, test of choice for valve problems
_____ Holter monitor	

d. Dye is injected during a cardiac catheterization; determines patency of coronary arteries and the presence of collateral circulation

e. Tourniquet placed on extremity and die injected into affected extremity; used to detect thrombi within the venous system

f. A miniature electrocardiogram (ECG) recorder; correlates normal daily activity with electrical function of the heart to determine whether activity causes abnormalities

13. List at least three interventions for the prevention of stasis ulcers for a patient at risk for the development of the condition.

14. A weight gain of _____ pounds in a 24-hour period signals edema.

15. When caring for a patient who is expressing unrelieved chest pain, which of the following medications should the nurse anticipate as most likely to be ordered by the physician?
    a. Demerol
    b. Nubain
    c. Narcan
    d. Morphine sulfate

16. When caring for a patient experiencing right-sided heart failure, the nurse must understand which of the following? Select all that apply.

    _____ Weakness in the ventricle has resulted in a reduction of cardiac output.

    _____ Valvular disease is a potential risk factor.

    _____ Pulmonary stenosis is an associated risk factor.

    _____ The heart has a reduction in contraction strength.

    _____ Pallor and clammy skin are common clinical manifestations.

 17. List the primary goals for treatment and/or management of heart failure. (*Hint:* See page 430 in your textbook.)

18. A patient has been diagnosed with a cardiac disorder in which separate impulses are causing contractions in the atrium and ventricles. Based on your knowledge, this patient is experiencing:
    a. complete heart block.
    b. premature ventricular contractions.
    c. ventricular fibrillation.
    d. ventricular tachycardia.
    e. atrial flutter.

19. Nifedipine (Procardia) has been prescribed for a patient who has a cardiac disorder. Based on your knowledge, to which of the following classifications does this medication belong?
    a. Calcium channel blockers
    b. Antidysrhythmics class I
    c. Beta blockers
    d. Potassium-sparing drugs

20. What impact can antihypertensive medications have on sexual function?

Exercise 2

 Virtual Hospital Activity

45 minutes

- Sign in to work at Pacific View Regional Hospital on the Medical-Surgical Floor for Period of Care 1. (*Note:* If you are already in the virtual hospital from a previous exercise, click on **Leave the Floor** and then on **Restart the Program** to get to the sign-in window.)
- From the Patient List, select Patricia Newman (Room 406).
- Click on **Get Report** and read the shift report.
- Click on **Go to Nurses' Station**.
- Click on **Chart**; then on **406**.
- Click on and review the **History and Physical** and **Nursing Admission**.

1. Patricia Newman has a 15-year history of hypertension. Identify the two factors that determine blood pressure.

2. The focus of management in the hypertensive patient is the _____ blood pressure.

3. _____ Hypertension is more common in women over age 55 than in men over age 55. (True/False)

4. Identify at least four significant health concerns in Patricia Newman's medical history.

5. Upon admission, Patricia Newman's blood pressure was _____.

6. As a result of her hypertension, Patricia Newman is at an increased risk for death related to

   damage to the _____, _____, and

   _____.

7. _____ Patricia Newman has secondary hypertension. (True/False)

8. Which of the following risk factors associated with hypertension apply to Patricia Newman? Select all that apply.

   _____ Dyslipidemia

   _____ Atherosclerosis

   _____ Diabetes mellitus

   _____ Cigarette smoking

   _____ Aging

   _____ Gender

   _____ Obesity

   _____ Sedentary lifestyle

9. For what complications is Patricia Newman at risk related to her hypertension? Why?

→ • Click on **Return to Nurses' Station**.
  • Click on the **Drug** icon and review the information for atenolol and chlorothiazide.

10. Patricia Newman takes atenolol 50 mg PO and chlorothiazide 500 mg PO daily to manage her hypertension. Identify the action or classification of each of these medications.

11. Explain the interrelationship between atenolol and chlorothiazide.

12. When administering atenolol to Patricia Newman, the nurse should be aware of which of the following?
    a. Atenolol is classified as a calcium channel blocker.
    b. The use of this medication may mask hypoglycemia.
    c. Atenolol is associated with an increase in lipid metabolism.
    d. Atenolol is used to increase cardiac output.

13. The normally recommended dosage of atenolol is _____ to _____ mg.

14. _____ Patricia Newman's prescribed dosage of atenolol is within recommended limits. (True/False)

15. Which of the following manifestations are side effects associated with atenolol? Select all that apply.

    _____ Cold extremities

    _____ Constipation

    _____ Diarrhea

    _____ Nausea

    _____ Headache

    _____ Impotence

16. Chlorothiazide is associated with excretion of which of the following electrolytes? Select all that apply.

_____ Sodium

_____ Phosphorus

_____ Potassium

_____ Zinc

_____ Calcium

_____ Magnesium

_____ Chloride

17. The normal potassium level is _____ to _____ mEq/L. (*Hint:* Consult your lab reference.)

18. Identify nursing considerations for Patricia Newman related to the medications prescribed to manage her hypertension.

→ • Click on **Return to Nurses' Station**.
  • Click on **406** at the bottom of your screen.
  • Inside the patient's room, click on **Take Vital Signs** and review.
  • Click on **Patient Care** and then on **Physical Assessment**.
  • Complete a systems assessment by clicking on the body system categories (yellow buttons) and subcategories (green buttons).

19. It is best to take Patricia Newman's blood pressure when she has been resting quietly for at

    least _____ minutes.

20. _____ Patricia Newman's blood pressure can be anticipated to be lowest right after a meal. (True/False)

21. _____ A review of Patricia Newman's physical assessment reflects the presence of early fluid retention. (True/False)

Exercise 3

Virtual Hospital Activity

30 minutes

- Sign in to work at Pacific View Regional Hospital on the Medical-Surgical Floor for Period of Care 1. (*Note:* If you are already in the virtual hospital from a previous exercise, click on **Leave the Floor** and then on **Restart the Program** to get to the sign-in window.)
- From the Patient List, select Piya Jordan (Room 403).
- Click on **Get Report** and read the shift report.
- Click on **Go to Nurses' Station**.
- Click on **Chart** and then on **403**.
- Click on and review the **History and Physical**.

1. What are some of the complaints that led Piya Jordan to seek medical treatment?

2. What significant factors are present in Piya Jordan's medical history?

3. Which of the following best describes Piya Jordan's cardiac disorder?
   a. Failure of the heart's ventricles to contract, causing a lack of cardiac output
   b. The occurrence of a flutter-like movement in the heart's atria
   c. The presence of episodes of tachycardia followed by periods of bradycardia
   d. The failure of the heart's atria and ventricles to contract with coordination

4. The presence of Piya Jordan's heart disorder increases her risk for which of the following?
   a. Clot formation
   b. Respiratory arrest
   c. Premature ventricular contractions
   d. Complete heart block

➡ • Click on and review the **Nursing Admission**.

5. _____ Piya Jordan is exhibiting the early signs of complications of her cardiovascular disorder. (True/False)

➡ • Click on **Return to Nurses' Station**.

• Click on the **Drug** icon and review information about the medications prescribed for Piya Jordan.

6. Before her current hospital admission, Piya Jordan was taking the medication listed below. Match each medication with its corresponding classification. (*Hint:* Consult your nursing drug guide as well.)

Medication	Action or Classification
_____ Digoxin 0.125 mg daily	a. Nonsteroidal antiinflammatory drug (NSAID)
_____ Warfarin 5 mg daily	b. Antiarrhythmic
_____ Celecoxib 200 mg every 12 hours	c. Anticoagulant

7. Do any of the medications prescribed for Piya Jordan present a possible concern for adverse reactions?

8. When administering these medications to Piya Jordan, the nurse must be aware of any

potential adverse interactions between _____ and

_____.

9. The normal dosage range for digoxin administered orally is _____ mg to _____ mg.

10. _____ The dosage of digoxin prescribed for Piya Jordan is higher than normally recommended ranges. (True/False)

11. When preparing to administer digoxin, the nurse must ensure that the apical pulse is greater

than _____.

→ • Click on **Return to Nurses' Station**.
  • Click on **403** at the bottom of the screen.
  • Click on **Take Vital Signs** and review.
  • Click on **Patient Care** and then on **Physical Assessment**.
  • Click on **Chest**; then on **Cardiovascular.**

12. Discuss any abnormal findings of the cardiac assessment.

Care of Patients with Neurologic Disorders

 Reading Assignment: The Neurologic System (Chapter 22)
Care of Patients with Head and Spinal Cord Injuries
(Chapter 23)
Care of Patients with Disorders of the Brain (Chapter 24)

Patient: Goro Oishi, Skilled Nursing Floor, Room 505

Objectives:

1. Become familiar with techniques for assessment of the nervous system.

2. Describe diagnostic tests used to evaluate functioning of the nervous system.

3. Compare and contrast the various signs and symptoms of the common problems experienced by patients with nervous system disorders.

4. Describe the pathophysiology of increasing intracranial pressure (ICP).

5. Recall the signs and symptoms (from early to late) of increasing ICP.

Exercise 1

 Writing Activity

35 minutes

1. The central nervous system is composed of the _____ and

_____ _____.

2. Discuss the interaction between the peripheral nervous system (PNS) and the central nervous system (CNS).

3. List at least four nervous system changes associated with aging.

4. Match each of the following diagnostic tests with its correct description.

Diagnostic Test	Description
_____ Lumbar puncture	a. Used to visualize soft tissue by use of an electromagnet to detect radiofrequency pulses produced by alignment of hydrogen protons in the magnetic field
_____ Electroencephalography (EEG)	
_____ Electromyography (EMG)	
_____ Computed axial tomography (CAT scan)	b. Used to assess cerebral spinal fluid (CSF) by means of a sterile puncture into the arachnoid space
_____ Cerebral angiography	c. Allows visualization of the brain from many different angles
_____ Magnetic resonance imaging (MRI)	d. Assesses for cell death; radioactive material is administered providing differing color in areas of cellular activity
_____ Positron emission tomography (PET)	
	e. Used to detect brain wave patterns
	f. Used to measure electrical activity in skeletal muscle during rest and activity
	g. Visualizes structures of the cerebral arteries by the injection of a radiopaque liquid through the common carotid artery

5. _____ An increase in systolic blood pressure accompanied by a decrease in diastolic blood pressure is a manifestation of decreasing ICP. (True/False)

6. _____ The patient who exhibits extension of the legs and internal rotation and adduction of the arms with the elbows bent upward has likely experienced damage to the brain's cortex. (True/False)

7. _____ The nurse may assign assistive personnel to take the vital signs of an unconscious patient. (True/False)

8. A nurse developed a plan of care for a patient diagnosed with a neurologic disorder. Which of the following nursing diagnoses is the highest priority?
   a. Ineffective breathing pattern related to neurologic disruption of respirations
   b. Knowledge deficit related to disorder
   c. Impaired physical mobility related to weakness and fatigue
   d. Self-care deficit related to neurologic impairment

9. The new term used to refer to quadriplegia is _____.

10. A nurse performs a neurologic assessment on a patient and notes the patient is having difficulty swallowing. Which of the following terms should the nurse record in the patient's record?
    a. Dysuria
    b. Hemiplegia
    c. Hemiparesis
    d. Dysphagia

11. A nurse is preparing to initiate a schedule for bladder training for a patient who has a neurogenic bladder. How often should the patient be encouraged to void?
    a. Every hour
    b. Every 2 hours
    c. Every 4 hours
    d. Whenever the patient indicates the sensation of fullness

12. As the nurse completes a neurologic assessment, the patient moans his answers and has only slight responses to vigorous stimulation. Which of the terms below can best be used to describe this patient?
    a. Comatose
    b. Stuporous
    c. Obtunded
    d. Lethargic
    e. Confused

13. A patient has experienced periorbital fractures with ecchymoses behind the ear. This is

    termed _____ _____.

14. The head of the bed for a patient who has experienced a head injury should be elevated

    to _____ degrees.

15. A patient who experienced a head injury is at risk for the development of deep vein thrombosis (DVT). List at least three interventions that can be implemented to reduce the risk for DVT. (*Hint:* See pages 416-418 in your textbook.)

Exercise 2

 Virtual Hospital Activity

 30 minutes

- Sign in to work at Pacific View Regional Hospital on the Skilled Nursing Floor for Period of Care 1. (*Note:* If you are already in the virtual hospital from a previous exercise, click on **Leave the Floor** and then on **Restart the Program** to get to the sign-in window.)
- From the Patient List, select Goro Oishi (Room 505).
- Click on **Get Report** and read the shift report.
- Click on **Go to Nurses' Station**.
- Click on **Chart** and then on **505**.
- Click on and review the **Nursing Admission** and **History and Physical**.

1. What is Goro Oishi's diagnosis?

2. What is Goro Oishi's prognosis?

3. List the initial complaints that led Goro Oishi to seek medical care.

4. Which of the following risk factors associated with a cerebrovascular accident does Goro Oishi have? Select all that apply.

_____ Hypertension

_____ Cigarette smoking

_____ Hyperlipidemia

_____ Diabetes

_____ Excessive alcohol intake

_____ Obesity

_____ Use of cocaine or other recreational drugs

_____ Heart disease

_____ Sedentary lifestyle

_____ History of transient ischemic attacks

_____ Age 65 years or older

_____ Male gender

5. There are different types of cerebrovascular accidents (CVAs). Match each of the following types of CVA with its correct description.

Type of CVA	**Description**
_____ Cerebral thrombosis	a. Traveling blood clot, fat, bacteria, or tissue debris that lodges in a vessel, occluding it
_____ Embolus	b. Formation of a blood clot in a cerebral artery
_____ Intracerebral hemorrhage	c. Occurs when a blood vessel ruptures and leaks blood into brain tissue or an aneurysm leaks or ruptures

→ • Click on **Return to Nurses' Station**; then click on **505** at the bottom of your screen.
  • Review the Initial Observations.
  • Click on **Take Vital Signs** and review the findings.

6. To reduce ICP, the physician has ordered the head of Goro Oishi's bed to be elevated only

   to _____ degrees.

7. Record Goro Oishi's vital signs. (*Note:* Answers will vary depending on the exact time vital
   signs are taken.)

→ • Click on **Patient Care** and then on **Physical Assessment**.
  • Complete a systems assessment by clicking on the body system categories (yellow buttons)
    and subcategories (green buttons).

8. Goro Oishi's assessment reflects a score of _____ on the Glasgow Coma Scale.

9. The Glasgow Coma Scale (GCS) assesses _____ opening,

   _____ response, and _____ response.

10. _____ A GCS score of 5 or below reflects a totally comatose patient. (True/False)

11. Goro Oishi's assessment reflects the presence of decerebrate posturing. How does this type
    of posturing appear?
    a. Extension of the legs and internal rotation and adduction of the arms with the elbows
       bent upward
    b. Stiff extension of the arms and flexion of the wrists
    c. Flexion of the legs and external rotation of the arms
    d. None of the above

12. Decerebrate posturing indicates damage to the _____ or _____.

13. Goro Oishi's brainstem function can be assessed by checking the doll's eye reflex. What
    does this examination entail? How would you expect Goro Oishi's eyes to react?

14. _____ Goro Oishi's pupils can be best described as "pinpoint." (True/False)

15. Review Goro Oishi's pupillary responses and list three potential causes for them. (*Hint:* See page 489 in your textbook.)

16. _____ Goro Oishi's blood pressure indicates increasing ICP. (True/False)

→ • Click on **Chart** and then on **505**.
  • Click on and review the **Physician's Orders**.

17. What orders concerning Goro Oishi's blood pressure have been left by the physician?

9

Care of Patients with Gastrointestinal Disorders

👓 **Reading Assignment:** The Gastrointestinal System (Chapter 28)

Care of Patients with Disorders of the Upper Gastrointestinal System (Chapter 29)

Care of Patients with Disorders of the Lower Gastrointestinal System (Chapter 30)

Patients: Piya Jordan, Medical-Surgical Floor, Room 403

Clarence Hughes, Medical-Surgical Floor, Room 404

Objectives:

1. Identify three major causative factors in the development of disorders of the gastrointestinal (GI) system.

2. Explain three measures to prevent the development of disorders of the gastrointestinal system.

3. Describe the assessment of a patient with a gastrointestinal disorder.

4. Describe the pathophysiology, diagnostic testing, clinical manifestations, and care of patients with selected gastrointestinal disorders.

Exercise 1

Writing Activity

30 minutes

1. The functions of the digestive tract are _____, _____,

_____, and _____.

2. When the nurse assesses the abdomen for bowel sounds, the _____ of the stethoscope must be used.

3. The normal frequency of bowel sounds is _____ to _____ in a 1-minute period of time.

4. When caring for a patient who has had an esophagogastroduodenoscopy performed, the nurse should include which of the following in the plan of care?
   a. Monitor stools for at least 2 days for the passage of white stools.
   b. Administer prescribed laxatives.
   c. Encourage fluid intake to flush the patient's system.
   d. Ensure NPO until gag reflex returns.

5. Which of the following events can increase the body's nutritional needs? Select all that apply.

   _____ Infection

   _____ Fever

   _____ Rest

   _____ Stress

   _____ Trauma

6. List at least three factors that promote obesity.

7. To reduce the risk for aspiration after a tube feeding, the nurse should keep the head of the bed elevated for how long?
   a. 15 minutes
   b. 30 minutes
   c. 1 hour
   d. 90 minutes

8. If undigested fat is present in the stool, the stool will _____

   _____.

9. A patient undergoes a gastric surgical procedure. During the procedure, the end of the stomach is connected to the duodenum. Based on your knowledge, you recognize the patient has had a:
   a. total gastrectomy.
   b. modified gastrectomy.
   c. Billroth I procedure.
   d. Billroth II procedure.

10. Using the table below, compare and contrast gastric ulcers and duodenal ulcers.

	Gastric Ulcer	Duodenal Ulcer
Location		
Population		
Manifestations		

11. Most ulcers are caused by _____.

12. Match each of the following gastrointestinal disorders with its correct description.

Gastrointestinal Disorder	**Description**
_____ Gastroesophageal reflux disease (GERD)	a. The presence of herniations in the muscular layers of the colon
_____ Gastritis	b. An inflammatory condition of the gastrointestinal tract causing a cobblestone-like appearance in the mucosa
_____ Irritable bowel syndrome (IBS)	
_____ Ulcerative colitis	c. Alteration in bowel elimination, abdominal pain and bloating, and absence of detectable organic disease
_____ Crohn's disease	
_____ Diverticulosis	d. The presence of abscesses on the colon mucosa and submucosa, causing drainage and sloughing and subsequent ulcerations
	e. The backflow of stomach acid into the esophagus
	f. Inflammation of the lining of the stomach

13. Match each of the following drugs with its correct use or action.

Drug	Use or Action
_____ Diphenoxylate HCl (Lomotil)	a. Provides protective barrier over ulcer surface
_____ Metoclopramide (Reglan)	b. Antiinfective used to manage inflammatory bowel disease (IBD)
_____ Sulfasalazine (Azulfidine)	
_____ Sucralfate (Carafate)	c. Decreases intestinal motility
_____ Cimetidine (Tagamet)	d. Suppress acid secretion by blocking H_2 receptors on parietal cells
	e. Increases the speed of gastric emptying into the small intestine

14. List at least three potential clinical manifestations associated with constipation.

15. When providing care for a patient complaining of gas buildup, which of the following positions (if not contraindicated) may best assist the patient to expel the flatus?
    a. Trendelenburg
    b. Supine
    c. Prone
    d. Standing

16. _____ Hot drinks may create more abdominal gas. (True/False)

17. When providing care to a patient experiencing nausea or vomiting, the nurse knows that which of the following foods should be avoided during the first 24 hours? Select all that apply.

    _____ Plain hard candy

    _____ Cheese

    _____ Pudding

    _____ Citrus juice

    _____ Pear juice

    _____ Popsicles

18. Lactose intolerance is most common in _____.

Exercise 2

Virtual Hospital Activity

30 minutes

- Sign in to work at Pacific View Regional Hospital on the Medical-Surgical Floor for Period of Care 2. (*Note:* If you are already in the virtual hospital from a previous exercise, click on **Leave the Floor** and then on **Restart the Program** to get to the sign-in window.)
- From the Patient List, select Piya Jordan (Room 403).
- Click on **Get Report** and read the shift report.
- Click on **Go to Nurses' Station**.
- Click on **Chart**; then on **403**.
- Click on and review the **History and Physical**, **Diagnostic Reports**, and **Nursing Admission**.

1. Why did Piya Jordan initially seek care?

2. What was diagnosed after Piya Jordan's medical examination in the Emergency Department?

3. An intestinal obstruction can be caused by a mass as well as a number of other factors. List at least five other factors that can result in an intestinal obstruction.

4. The vomiting associated with an intestinal obstruction can lead to fluid and electrolyte

   imbalances and _____.

5. Intestinal obstructions can be classified as mechanical or nonmechanical. How do they differ? Which type of obstruction does Piya Jordan have?

6. Which of the following diagnostic tests were used to determine the underlying cause of Piya Jordan's condition? Select all that apply.

   _____   Computed tomography (CT) of abdomen

   _____   Kidney-ureter-bladder (KUB) scan

   _____   Chest x-ray

   _____   Electrocardiogram (ECG)

   _____   Endoscopy

   _____   Colonoscopy

→ •   Still in Piya Jordan's chart, click on and review the **Surgical Reports**.

7. What were the postoperative diagnoses?

8. Which of the following best describes the surgical procedure performed?
   a. Removal of the entire small intestine
   b. Removal of the entire large intestine
   c. Removal of the distal portion of the stomach and the small intestine
   d. Removal of a portion of the large intestine

9. It is possible Piya Jordan has adenocarcinoma. List at least six factors that can predispose an individual to this disease.

10. The portion of the intestine involved in Piya Jordan's obstruction is the

_____.

- Click on **Return to Nurses' Station**.
- Click on **403** at the bottom of the screen.
- Inside the patient's room, click on **Take Vital Signs**.
- Review the Initial Observations.
- Click on and review the **Clinical Alerts**.
- Click on **Patient Care** and then on **Nurse-Client Interactions**.
- Select and view the video titled **1115: Interventions—Nausea, Blood**. (*Note:* Check the virtual clock to see whether enough time has elapsed. You can use the fast-forward feature to advance the time by 2-minute intervals if the video is not yet available. Then click again on **Patient Care** and on **Nurse-Client Interactions** to refresh the screen.)

11. Based on your review of the shift report and the nurse's interaction with Piya Jordan, which care factors appear to be of the highest priority?

- Click on **Patient Care** and then on **Physical Assessment**.
- Complete a systems assessment by clicking on the body system categories (yellow buttons) and subcategories (green buttons).

12. Piya Jordan's assessment findings reflect the greatest potential for the development of postoperative complications in which of the following body systems?
    a. Respiratory system
    b. Renal system
    c. Integumentary system
    d. Reproductive system
    e. Neurologic system

13. Management and care of the patient who has had gastrointestinal surgery frequently includes the placement of a nasogastric (NG) tube. An NG tube has a variety of functions. Match each of the following functions with its correct description.

Function	**Description**
_____ Decompression	a. Irrigation of the stomach; used in cases of active bleeding, poisoning, or gastric dilation
_____ Feeding	
	b. Removal of secretions and gases from the gastrointestinal tract
_____ Compression	
	c. Internal application of pressure by means of an inflated balloon to prevent internal gastrointestinal hemorrhage
_____ Lavage	
	d. Installation of liquid supplements into the stomach

14. Piya Jordan has had an NG tube inserted for _____.

15. Discuss the responsibilities of the nurse concerning the care and management of Piya Jordan's NG tube.

 • Click on **EPR** and then on **Login**.
 • Select **403** for the Patient drop-down menu and **Intake and Output** from the Category drop-down menu.

16. Review the output from Piya Jordan's NG tube. What is the total amount of drainage from the tube since surgery?

17. _____ The absence of bowel sounds in Piya Jordan at this stage of her recovery is
abnormal. (True/False)

18. When the nurse performs the assessment of Piya Jordan's abdomen, in what order should
the steps be performed? Match each of the following assessment tools with its order of
occurrence.

Assessment Tool	Order of Occurrence
_____ Palpation	a. First
_____ Inspection	b. Second
_____ Percussion	c. Third
_____ Auscultation	d. Fourth

Exercise 3

  Virtual Hospital Activity

45 minutes

- Sign in to work at Pacific View Regional Hospital on the Medical-Surgical Floor for Period
  of Care 1. (*Note:* If you are already in the virtual hospital from a previous exercise, click on
  Leave the Floor and then on **Restart the Program** to get to the sign-in window.)
- From the Patient List, select Clarence Hughes (Room 404).
- Click on **Get Report** and read the shift report.
- Click on **Go to Nurses' Station**; then click on **404** at the bottom of the screen.
- Click on and review the **Clinical Alerts**.
- Click on **Patient Care** and then on **Nurse-Client Interactions**.
- Select and view the videos titled **0730: Assessment/Perception of Care** and
  0735: Empathy. (*Note:* Check the virtual clock to see whether enough time has elapsed.
  You can use the fast-forward feature to advance the time by 2-minute intervals if the video is
  not yet available. Then click again on **Patient Care** and then on **Nurse-Client Interactions**
  to refresh the screen.)
- Click on **Patient Care** and then on **Physical Assessment**.
- Complete head-to-toe systems assessment by clicking on the body system category (yellow
  buttons) and subcategories (green buttons).

1. What are the two primary complaints being voiced by Clarence Hughes?

2. Review the characteristics of the patient's last reported bowel movement.

3. The consistency of the stool is a reflection of its _____ content.

4. Stools can be _____, _____,

   _____, or _____.

5. Which of the following surgery-related events has the most bearing on Clarence Hughes'
   current state of constipation?
   a. Direct handling of the bowel during the operative procedure
   b. The onset of a paralytic ileus
   c. Postoperative edema at the site of the surgical intervention
   d. Administration of operative and postoperative medications

6. When visualizing Clarence Hughes' abdomen, the nurse should be looking for what?

7. _____ When evaluating Clarence Hughes' bowel sounds, the nurse can use the
   auditory characteristics of these sounds as clues to conditions within the bowel.
   (True/False)

8. During the abdominal assessment, the abdomen should be divided into four

   _____.

9. When evaluating the abdominal assessment, the nurse recognizes the presence of a dull
   sound with percussion as indicative of:
   a. air.
   b. the onset of a paralytic ileus.
   c. feces.
   d. bladder distention.

→ • Click on **Chart** and then on **404**.
  • Click on and review the **Nursing Admission** and **History and Physical**.

10. Clarence Hughes normally has a bowel movement _____.

11. Are Clarence Hughes' typical bowel habits normal for a patient of his age and gender?

12. A review of Clarence Hughes' medical history identifies which of the following to be potential underlying factors associated with the development of his constipation?
    a. Condition of his teeth
    b. Dietary intake
    c. Psychosocial factors
    d. Use of pharmacologic interventions to achieve a bowel movement
    e. History of bowel disorders
    f. None of the above

➡ • Click on **Return to Room 404**.
   • Click on **MAR** and then on **404**. Review the medications prescribed for Clarence Hughes.

13. Which of the medications prescribed for Clarence Hughes may promote constipation? Select all that apply. (*Hint:* If needed, click on the **Drug** icon for reference information.)

   _____ Docusate sodium

   _____ Celecoxib

   _____ Timolol maleate

   _____ Pilocarpine 1% ophthalmic solution

   _____ Enoxaparin

   _____ Promethazine hydrochloride

   _____ Magnesium hydroxide

   _____ Aluminum hydroxide with magnesium simethicone

   _____ Bisacodyl

   _____ Acetaminophen

   _____ Temazepam

   _____ Oxycodone with acetaminophen

14. _____ are agents that stimulate defecation, and

    _____ are strong laxatives that produce a watery stool.

15. Match each of the following laxative types with its correct description or action.

Type of Laxative	**Description or Action**
_____ Bulk-forming	a. An osmotic agent that draws water into the intestine to increase bulk and lubricate feces
_____ Lubricant	
_____ Saline	b. A synthetic or natural polysaccharide and cellulose derivative that absorbs water and increases stool volume, thus stimulating peristalsis
_____ Stimulant	
	c. Increases peristalsis by stimulating sensory nerve endings of the colonic epithelium or by irritation of the GI mucosa
	d. Provides a coating of the outer fecal mass, which makes the mass slippery and inhibits its ability to absorb fluid

16. Match each of the following laxatives with its appropriate classification. (*Note:* You will use some classifications more than once.)

Laxative	**Classification**
_____ Bran	a. Stimulant
_____ Colace	b. Bulk-forming laxative
_____ Magnesium hydroxide	c. Osmotic agent
_____ Bisacodyl	d. Lubricant laxative
_____ Dialose	
_____ Lactulose	

17. Which medications have been prescribed to manage Clarence Hughes' constipation?

Now let's prepare to administer medications for Clarence Hughes to manage his constipation.

- From the MAR, click on **Return to Room 404**.
- Click on **Medication Room**.
- Click on **Unit Dosage** and then on drawer **404**.
- Select **Magnesium hydroxide** and click on **Put Medication on Tray**.
- When finished with the storage area, click on **Close Drawer**.
- Click on **View Medication Room**.
- Now click on **Preparation** and choose the correct medication to administer. Click on **Prepare**.
- Click on **Next** and choose the correct patient to administer this medication to. Click on **Finish**.
- You can **Review Your Medications** and then on **Return to Medication Room** when ready.

18. The dosage of medication obtained was _____ mL.

19. The physician has also ordered a bisacodyl suppository for Clarence Hughes. This

   medication will act as a _____ to stimulate gastrointestinal

   _____.

20. If the bisacodyl suppository is administered, how long should Clarence Hughes attempt to retain it?
   a. 5-10 minutes
   b. 20-30 minutes
   c. 1-2 hours
   d. Overnight

LESSON 10

Musculoskeletal and Connective Tissue Disorders

👓 **Reading Assignment:** The Musculoskeletal System (Chapter 32)
Care of Patients with Musculoskeletal and Connective Tissue Disorders (Chapter 33)

Patients: Kathryn Doyle, Skilled Nursing Floor, Room 503
Harry George, Medical-Surgical Floor, Room 401
Clarence Hughes, Medical-Surgical Floor, Room 404

Objectives:

1. Recall the normal anatomy of the musculoskeletal system.
2. Identify the functions of the musculoskeletal system.
3. Describe the diagnostic tests and procedures used for assessing connective tissue diseases.
4. Discuss the drugs used to treat connective tissue diseases.
5. Describe the pathophysiology and treatment for selected disorders of the musculoskeletal system.

Exercise 1

Writing Activity

30 minutes

1. A patient who is taking steroids asks why long-term use may cause musculoskeletal disorders. Which of the following is correct?
   a. Steroids increase the rate of bone absorption.
   b. Long-term steroid use is associated with osteoporosis.
   c. Long-term steroid use is associated with increased ossification.
   d. Steroid use reduces calcium absorption.

2. When performing an assessment of the musculoskeletal system, a nurse must listen for a

   crackling sound known as _____.

3. List at least six age-related changes in connective tissue.

4. When preparing a patient for a C-reactive protein test, the nurse should include which of the following in the patient teaching?
   a. Advise the patient to fast for 8 hours before the test.
   b. Obtain a clean-catch midstream urine specimen.
   c. Restrict red meat intake the day before the test.
   d. Restrict fluids and food for 4 hours before the test.

5. What is the acronym used to signify management for sprains? What does each letter in the acronym stand for?

6. _____ Drug therapy can provide a cure for osteoarthritis. (True/False)

7. _____ To avoid addiction, patients with osteoarthritis should take medications only when pain is present. (True/False)

8. _____ Rheumatoid disorders affect women more frequently than men. (True/False)

9. The onset of rheumatoid arthritis is between _____ and _____ years of age.

10. Which of the following factors are associated with rheumatoid arthritis? Select all that apply.

_____ Autoimmune reaction

_____ Infectious agents

_____ Genetic predisposition

_____ Reproductive history

_____ Hormonal factors

_____ Breastfeeding

_____ History of osteoarthritis

11. Which of the following clinical manifestations are associated with rheumatoid arthritis? Select all that apply.

_____ Pain aggravated by movement

_____ Pain that eases within 20-30 minutes after rising in the morning

_____ Weakness

_____ Weight gain

_____ Bilateral joint changes

_____ Muscle aches and tenderness

12. Gout is a systemic disease characterized by deposits of _____

_____ in the joints and other body tissues.

13. Which of the following factors are associated with gout? Select all that apply.

_____ Genetic links

_____ Malnutrition

_____ Alcohol consumption

_____ Hypouricemia

_____ Thiazide diuretics

14. When treating an acute episode of gout, the physician might prescribe which of the following medications?
    a. Colchicine
    b. Indomethacin
    c. Corticotrophin
    d. Sulfa compounds
    e. Allopurinol

15. When a nurse is planning a diet for a patient with gout, which of the following foods should be excluded? Select all that apply.

_____ Leafy green vegetables

_____ Gravy

_____ Sardines

_____ Organ meats

_____ Citrus fruits

Exercise 2

Virtual Hospital Activity

30 minutes

- Sign in to work at Pacific View Regional Hospital on the Skilled Nursing Unit for Period of Care 1. (*Note:* If you are already in the virtual hospital from a previous exercise, click on **Leave the Floor** and then on **Restart the Program** to get to the sign-in window.)
- From the Patient List, select Kathryn Doyle (Room 503).
- Click on **Get Report** and read the shift report.
- Click on **Go to Nurses' Station**.
- Click on **Chart** and then on **503**.
- Click on and review the **History and Physical** and **Nursing Admission**.

1. Why has Kathryn Doyle been admitted to the Skilled Nursing Unit?

2. Which of the following items in her medical history place Kathryn Doyle at an increased risk for a fracture? Select all that apply.

_____ 15-year history of osteoporosis

_____ Hysterectomy

_____ Tonsillectomy

_____ Malnutrition

_____ Family history of cardiovascular disease

_____ Sedentary lifestyle

3. _____ Kathryn Doyle's fracture can be described as pathologic. (True/False)

→ • Now click on and review the **Physician's Orders** and **Consultations**.

4. At this point in her recovery, Kathryn Doyle's bone healing can best be described as which of the following?
   a. Hematoma
   b. Granulation tissue
   c. Callus
   d. Ossification
   e. Consolidation and remodeling

5. Kathryn Doyle has had an ORIF. What does *ORIF* stand for?

6. When performing an ORIF, the surgeon may use _____,

   _____, _____, or

   _____ to realign and secure the fracture.

→ • Click on **Return to Nurses' Station**.
   • Click on **503** at the bottom of the screen.
   • Inside the patient's room, click on **Take Vital Signs**.
   • Click on and review the **Clinical Alerts**.
   • Click on **Patient Care** and then on **Physical Assessment**.
   • Complete a systems assessment by clicking on the body system categories (yellow buttons) and subcategories (green buttons).

7. What are Kathryn Doyle's vital signs? (*Note:* Findings may vary depending on the exact time vital signs are taken.)

8. Kathryn Doyle is using a(n) _____ pillow.

9. What precautions should be implemented for Kathryn Doyle in regard to her specialized leg pillow?

10. Which of the following positions are contraindicated for Kathryn Doyle? Select all that apply.

   _____ Lying on operative side

   _____ Crossing legs at the knees

   _____ Crossing legs at the ankles

   _____ Sitting in high chairs

   _____ Sitting in low chairs

11. Adequate nutrition is necessary to promote healing. Based on Kathryn Doyle's weight of 105 pounds, how much protein should her diet contain? (*Hint:* See page 743 in your textbook.)
   a. 10.5 g
   b. 37 g
   c. 47 g
   d. 50 g
   e. 75 g

→ • Click on **MAR** and then on **503**.
   • Review the medications ordered for Kathryn Doyle.

12. _____ Kathryn Doyle regularly takes medications that increase her risk for osteoporosis. (True/False)

13. The following medications have been ordered for Kathryn Doyle. Match each medication with its correct classification or usage. (*Hint:* If you need help, return to the patient's room and click on the **Drug** icon to access the Drug Guide.)

   Medication

   _____ Calcium citrate

   _____ Ferrous sulfate

   _____ Docusate sodium

   _____ Ibuprofen

   _____ Oxycodone

   _____ Acetaminophen

   Classification or Use

   a. Iron preparation; hematinic

   b. Stool softener

   c. Nonsteroidal antiinflammatory (NSAID); antipyretic; nonnarcotic analgesic

   d. Antipyretic; nonnarcotic analgesic

   e. Antiosteoporotic; antacid; phosphate adsorbent

   f. Schedule II narcotic analgesic; opiate derivative

14. Kathryn Doyle's physician has prescribed calcium supplements to manage her osteoporosis. Which of the following nursing implementations should be observed when administering this medication? Select all that apply.

_____ Administer medication with juice before meals to promote absorption.

_____ Administer medication with water 2 to 4 hours after meals.

_____ Monitor patient for signs of hypercalcemia.

_____ Monitor patient's blood pressure.

_____ Administer medication 1 hour after meals.

15. What relationship does the nurse need to be aware of between the calcium citrate and the ferrous sulfate? How will this relationship affect the manner of administration?

Exercise 3

 Virtual Hospital Activity

 30 minutes

- Sign in to work at Pacific View Regional Hospital on the Medical-Surgical Floor for Period of Care 1. (*Note:* If you are already in the virtual hospital from a previous exercise, click on **Leave the Floor** and then on **Restart the Program** to get to the sign-in window.)
- From the Patient List, select Harry George (Room 401).
- Click on **Get Report** and read the shift report.
- Click on **Go to Nurses' Station**.
- Click on **Chart** and then on **401**.
- Click on and review the **Nursing Admission**.

1. What factors in Harry George's medical and social history place him at risk for the development of osteomyelitis?

2. Which of the following clinical manifestations are associated with osteomyelitis? Select all that apply.

_____ Generalized pain

_____ Erythema in surrounding tissues

_____ Severe pain at the site

_____ Elevated temperature

_____ Chills

→ • Click on and review the **Laboratory Reports** and **Diagnostic Reports**.

3. Which of the following tests were ordered specifically to confirm the diagnosis of osteomyelitis? Select all that apply.

_____ Complete blood count (CBC)

_____ Urinalysis

_____ Albumin levels

_____ Hemoglobin A_{1C}

_____ Blood alcohol levels

_____ Folic acid levels

_____ Bone scan

_____ X-ray of left foot

_____ Chest x-ray

4. Which of Harry George's laboratory values are abnormal? Select all that apply.

_____ Red blood cell count (RBC)

_____ White blood cell count (WBC)

_____ Hemoglobin

_____ Hematocrit

_____ Platelets

_____ Neutrophil segs

_____ Neutrophil bands

_____ Lymphocytes

_____ Monocytes

_____ Eosinophils

_____ Basophils

5. Which of the following statements concerning Harry George's erythrocyte sedimentation rate (ESR) is correct?
   a. The ESR is decreased as a result of the infection.
   b. The ESR is increased as a result of the infection.
   c. Harry George's diabetes suppresses the ESR value.
   d. Patients with diabetes have an natural elevation in ESR.

6. Discuss the results of Harry George's x-ray and bone scan.

7. _____ has been identified as the pathogen responsible for Harry George's infection.

8. _____ Harry George also has tested positive for septicemia. (True/False)

➤ • Click on and review the **Physician's Orders**.

9. In addition to medications, what has been ordered to manage Harry George's osteomyelitis?

10. What consultations have been ordered to assist in the treatment of Harry George's osteomyelitis?

- Click on **Return to Nurses' Station**.
- Click on **401** at the bottom of the screen.
- Read the Initial Observations.
- Click on and review the **Clinical Alerts**.
- Click on **Take Vital Signs**.

11. Record Harry George's vital signs. (*Note:* Findings may vary depending on the exact time vital signs are taken.)

12. Which of Harry George's vital signs are consistent with the presence of an infection?

- Click on **Patient Care** and then on **Physical Assessment**.
- Complete a head-to-toe assessment by clicking on the body system categories (yellow buttons) and subcategories (green buttons).

13. What findings from the assessment of Harry George's lower extremities are consistent with the diagnosis of osteomyelitis?

• Click on **MAR** and then on **401**.
 • Review Harry George's ordered medications.

14. Which of the following medications have been ordered to manage Harry George's infection? Select all that apply.

_____ Gentamycin 20 mg IV

_____ Thiamine 100 mg PO/IM

_____ Cefotaxime 2 g IV

_____ Phenytoin sodium 100 mg IV

_____ Aluminum hydroxide with magnesium 30 mL

15. Once administered, the analgesic will take effect in:
   a. 10-15 minutes.
   b. 30-45 minutes.
   c. 1 hour.
   d. 90 minutes.

16. Harry George can expect effects of the medication to last:
   a. 2-3 hours.
   b. 4-5 hours.
   c. 6-7 hours.
   d. 8-9 hours.

Exercise 4

 Virtual Hospital Activity

 30 minutes

 • Sign in to work at Pacific View Regional Hospital on the Medical-Surgical Floor for Period of Care 1. (*Note:* If you are already in the virtual hospital form a previous exercise, click on **Leave the Floor** and then on **Restart the Program** to get to the sign-in window.)
 • From the Patient List, select Clarence Hughes (Room 404).
 • Click on **Get Report** and read the shift report.
 • Click on **Go to Nurses' Station**
 • Click on **Chart** and then on **404**.
 • Inside the chart, click on and review the **History and Physical**, **Nursing Admission**, and **Physician's Notes**.

1. Why has Clarence Hughes been admitted to the hospital?

2. Clarence Hughes has a degenerative joint disease known as _____.

3. Which of the following populations are at an increased risk for the development of osteoarthritis? Select all that apply.

   _____ Small-framed patients

   _____ Obese patients

   _____ Older patients

   _____ Individuals whose occupations require repetitive joint movements

   _____ Women of childbearing age

   _____ Patients with diabetes

4. Which joints are most likely involved in osteoarthritis?

5. According to Clarence Hughes' assessment data, he has a history of an arthroscopy. Which of the following statements concerning this procedure is most correct?
   a. Arthroscopy involves obtaining a specimen of muscle tissue for study.
   b. Arthroscopy allows the visualization of the joint cavity.
   c. After arthroscopy there is no need to limit activity.
   d. Arthroscopy provides a definitive diagnosis for inflammatory connective tissue diseases.

6. Which of the following clinical manifestations are associated with osteoarthritis?
   a. Joint pain in the morning upon arising
   b. Bilateral joint involvement
   c. Joint enlargement
   d. Systemic involvement

7. Clarence Hughes has been taking celecoxib 100 mg PO BID to manage his condition. Which of the following correctly describe this medication? Select all that apply.

   _____ Antiinflammatory

   _____ Used to manage allergic conditions

   _____ Inhibits platelet aggregation

   _____ Antipyretic

   _____ Analgesic

➜ • Click on and review the **Surgical Reports**.

  8. What surgical procedure was completed to manage Clarence Hughes' condition?

  9. A joint replacement is avoided in patients younger than 50 years. (True/False)

➜ • Click on **Return to Nurses' Station** and then on **404** at the bottom of the screen.
  • Inside the patient's room, click on **Take Vital Signs**.
  • Now click on and review the **Initial Observations** and **Clinical Alerts**.
  • Click on **Patient Care** and then on **Physical Assessment**. Complete a systems assessment.

10. _____ Clarence Hughes' vital signs are within normal limits. (True/False)

11. What care needs for Clarence Hughes are highest in priority?

12. Which of the following interventions may be used to assist Clarence Hughes in the management of his postoperative pain? Select all that apply.

_____ Heating pad

_____ Massage

_____ Relaxation techniques

_____ Analgesics

_____ Imagery

13. _____ The physician has ordered Clarence Hughes to remain in bed for the first postoperative day. (True/False)

14. During the postoperative assessment, the nurse must remain on alert for the development of postoperative complications. List at least three potential complications for the patient who has had joint replacement surgery.

15. Which medication prescribed by the physician is intended to manage Clarence Hughes' pain?
    a. Acetaminophen 650 mg PO every 6 hours
    b. Temazepam 15 mg PO
    c. Oxycodone with acetaminophen 1-2 tablets PO every 4 hours
    d. Enoxaparin 30 mg subQ every 12 hours

LESSON 11

Care of Patients with Urinary Disorders

Reading Assignment: The Urinary System (Chapter 34)
Care of Patients with Disorders of the Urinary System
(Chapter 35)

Patient: William Jefferson, Skilled Nursing Floor, Room 501

Objectives:

1. Identify the clinical manifestations of common urinary disorders.
2. Discuss diagnostic tests used for urinary disorders.
3. Discuss key terms associated with the urinary system.
4. Identify potential causes of urinary disorders.

Exercise 1

 Writing Activity

 30 minutes

1. The waste products of urine include _____,

_____, and _____.

2. Match each key term with its corresponding definition.

Term	Definition
_____ Micturition	a. Difficult or painful urination
_____ Dysuria	b. That which is left in the bladder after voiding; related to poor muscle tone or partial obstruction
_____ Oliguria	c. Diminished, scant amounts of urine
_____ Anuria	d. The process of emptying the bladder
_____ Polyuria	e. The absence of urine
_____ Residual urine	f. The production of an excess of urine
_____ Nocturia	g. Urination at nighttime

3. The kidneys increase absorption of sodium in response to:
   a. aldosterone.
   b. antidiuretic hormone.
   c. atrial natriuretic hormone.
   d. renin.
   e. calcitriol.

4. Which of the following diagnostic tests may be used to examine the interior of the bladder?
   a. Cystoscopy
   b. Urethral pressure study
   c. Magnetic resonance imaging (MRI)
   d. Renal ultrasonography

5. Which of the following should be included in the teaching for a patient scheduled for a renal biopsy? Select all that apply.

   _____ The test requires the patient to be status nothing by mouth (NPO) for at least 8 to 10 hours before the procedure.

   _____ After the procedure, the patient will need to be on bedrest for 6 to 24 hours.

   _____ Heavy lifting should be avoided for 2 weeks after the procedure.

   _____ It is normal for the patient to experience bright red bleeding after the procedure for the first 2 days.

   _____ The procedure will only take 10 minutes.

6. Bright yellow urine may be associated with which of the following factors?
   a. Medication therapy
   b. Vitamin therapy
   c. The presence of bilirubin
   d. Reduced fluid intake

7. A delay in starting the stream of urine that may be related to partial obstruction is called

_____.

8. Urine output should be at least _____ mL per hour.

9. _____ The most common cause of hospital-acquired infections are urinary catheters. (True/False)

10. Name at least three drinks and substances that should be avoided in patients experiencing bladder control issues.

11. A patient has a catheter placed directly into the pelvis of the kidney to promote drainage of urine. Based on your knowledge, what type of device has been used?
   a. Urethral catheter
   b. Foley catheter
   c. Suprapubic catheter
   d. Urethral stint
   e. Nephrostomy tube

12. Which of the following foods are associated with a "healthy bladder"? Select all that apply.

_____ Lettuce

_____ Carrots

_____ Legumes

_____ Broccoli

_____ Cabbage

13. Identify at least three potential causes of acute renal failure (ARF).

14. A patient presents with fever, chills, flank pain, and marked hypertension. The history reveals recent "strep throat." Based on your knowledge, what diagnosis do you anticipate?
    a. Acute renal failure
    b. Acute glomerulonephritis
    c. Renal stenosis
    d. Pyelonephritis

15. A patient presents with recurring uric acid renal stones. What intervention is indicated to reduce future incidence of this type of stone?
    a. Avoid spinach, chard, and chocolate.
    b. Limit intake of protein-containing foods.
    c. Decrease intake of purine sources.
    d. Reduce sodium intake.

Exercise 2

 Virtual Hospital Activity

 30 minutes

- Sign in to work at Pacific View Regional Hospital on the Skilled Nursing Floor for Period of Care 1. (*Note:* If you are already in the virtual hospital from a previous exercise, click on **Leave the Floor** and then on **Restart the Program** to get to the sign-in window.)
- From the Patient List, select William Jefferson (Room 501).
- Click on **Get Report** and read the shift report.
- Click on **Go to Nurses' Station**.
- Click on **Chart** and then on **501**.
- Click on and review the **History and Physical**, **Nursing Admission**, and **Nurse's Notes**.

1. What was William Jefferson's chief complaint at the time of admission?

2. What illnesses are of interest in William Jefferson's past medical history?

3. One of the first signs of cystitis or urinary tract infection in the older adult is which of the following?
   a. Elevated temperature
   b. Flank pain
   c. Confusion
   d. Nausea
   e. Dysuria

4. Which of the following factors associated with aging may have contributed to the onset of William Jefferson's urinary tract infection? Select all that apply.

   _____   Reduced hormone levels

   _____   Nocturia

   _____   Residual urine

   _____   Hypertrophy of the prostate gland

   _____   Reduced secretion of renin

5. The causative agent identified in William Jefferson's urinary tract infection is

   _____.

→ • Click on and review the **Physician's Notes** and **Physician's Orders**.

6. Listed below are the medications prescribed by William Jefferson's physician. Match each medication with its correct description or action.

   Medication

   _____   Hydrochlorothiazide

   _____   Metformin

   _____   Rosiglitazone

   _____   Enalapril

   _____   Atenolol

   _____   Rivastigmine

   _____   Ibuprofen

   _____   Ciprofloxacin

   Description or Action

   a. Antihyperglycemic agent; decreases absorption of glucose, improves insulin sensitivity

   b. Nonnarcotic analgesic

   c. Antihypertensive agent, ACE inhibitor

   d. Antibiotic

   e. Antihypertensive agent, beta-1-adrenergic blocker

   f. Enhances cholinergic function

   g. Antihypertensive, diuretic-containing agent

   h. Antidiabetic, hypoglycemic agent; increases glucose utilization in skeletal muscles

7. A _____ medication is one considered potentially harmful to the kidneys.

8. Review William Jefferson's listing of prescribed medications. _____ is considered potentially harmful to kidney function.

9. When administering medications that are potentially nephrotoxic, what intervention can be implemented to reduce harm to the kidneys? What populations may not be suitable for implementing this intervention?

10. When administering ciprofloxacin to William Jefferson, the nurse is aware that the most common side effect experienced by patients taking the medication is which of the following?
    a. Dry mouth
    b. Nausea
    c. Ringing in the ears
    d. Abdominal pain

→ • Click on **Return to Nurses' Station** and then on **501** on the bottom of your screen.
  • Inside the patient's room, click on **Take Vital Signs**.
  • Click on **Patient Care** and then on **Physical Assessment**.
  • Complete a systems assessment by clicking on the body system categories (yellow buttons) and subcategories (green buttons).

11. _____ William Jefferson's vital signs are consistent with an ongoing infection. (True/False)

12. William Jefferson's assessment indicates the presence of nocturia. Which of the following is most likely responsible for this occurrence?
    a. A partial obstruction of the urethra
    b. A reduced ability of the kidney to concentrate urine
    c. Increased fluid intake
    d. Prescribed medications

→ • Click on **EPR** and then on **Login**.
  • Select **501** from the Patient drop-down menu and **Intake and Output** from the Category drop-down menu.

13. During his hospitalization, William Jefferson has been voiding quantities between

    _____ mL and _____ mL with each voiding.

14. The bladder is signaled to void when it contains approximately how much urine?
    a. 50-75 mL
    b. 75-125 mL
    c. 125-150 mL
    d. 150-200 mL

15. Calculate William Jefferson's intake and output for the 24-hour period beginning at 1900 on Sunday and ending Monday at 1859.

16. _____ William Jefferson's intake and output reflect fluid retention for the period specified in the previous question. (True/False)

17. Recommended fluid intake to maintain urologic system health is:
    a. 750-1000 mL/day.
    b. 1000-1500 mL/day.
    c. 1500-2000 mL/day.
    d. 2000-2500 mL/day.

Care of Patients with Endocrine Disorders

 Reading Assignment: The Endocrine System (Chapter 36)

Care of Patients with Diabetes and Hypoglycemia (Chapter 38)

Patient: Henry George, Medical-Surgical Floor, Room 401

Objectives:

1. Compare and contrast the different types of diabetes.
2. Discuss factors that influence the development of diabetes.
3. Review information concerning the types of insulin.

Exercise 1

Writing Activity

30 minutes

1. Match each of the following characteristics with the corresponding type of diabetes. Some types will be used more than once.

Characteristics	Type of Diabetes
_____ New patients are usually over 30 years of age and most are obese	a. Type 1 diabetes mellitus
_____ Appears early in life	b. Type 2 diabetes mellitus
_____ Occurs only during pregnancy	c. Gestational diabetes
_____ Rarely associated with ketoacidosis	d. Prediabetes
_____ Associated with obesity	
_____ Glucose levels are between those of people without diabetes and those with diabetes	
_____ Little endogenous insulin produced	

149

2. Which of the following are risk factors for the development of type 2 diabetes mellitus? Select all that apply.

_____ Underweight

_____ Sedentary lifestyle

_____ Age 30 and younger

_____ History of delivering infant weighing more than 10 pounds

_____ African American

_____ Latin American/Hispanic

3. _____% of the total population in the United States has diabetes mellitus.

4. Classic signs of diabetes include _____,

_____, and _____.

5. Insulin is a hormone produced by the _____ in the

_____.

6. Normal fasting serum glucose levels are between _____ and _____ mg/L. (*Hint:* Consult your lab reference.)

7. _____ Type 2 diabetes mellitus may be controlled by diet and exercise. (True/False)

8. _____ When preparing to mix insulin, cloudy insulin should be drawn into the syringe first. (True/False)

9. _____ Older adult patients experience hypoglycemia more quickly than do younger people. (True/False)

10. While at home, a patient begins to experience hypoglycemia. If the patient is able to swallow, which of the following choices could be consumed to manage the condition? Select all that apply.

_____ 2 cups of orange juice

_____ 1/2 cup of 2% or skim milk

_____ 1 can of regular soda

_____ 6 or 7 Life Savers

_____ 1 small box of raisins

11. Match each of the following types of insulin with its correct onset of action after administration.

Type of Insulin	**Onset of Action**
_____ Lantus	a. 15 minutes
_____ Humalog	b. 30 minutes
_____ NPH	c. 2-4 hours
_____ Regular	d. 1.5 hours

12. A patient with diabetes is planning to go bowling. Which of the following should be included in the patient's plans?
   a. Ingest 5 g of simple carbohydrates just before engaging in the activity.
   b. Ingest 10 g of simple carbohydrates 1 hour before engaging in the activity.
   c. Ingest 5 g of simple carbohydrates during a break in the activity.
   d. Ingest 5 g of simple carbohydrates after the first 30 minutes and at 30-minute intervals during the continued activity.

13. Humalog mix 75/25 was administered to a patient at 0900. At what time is the patient at the greatest risk for hypoglycemia?
   a. Between 0900 and 1100
   b. Between 1000 and 1300
   c. At bedtime
   d. In 24 hours

14. Which of the following should be incorporated into foot care for a patient with diabetes? Select all that apply.

   _____ Check feet daily.

   _____ Use heating pads instead of electric blankets for discomforts of the feet and legs.

   _____ Remove corns and calluses weekly.

   _____ Wear shoes without stockings to promote ventilation.

   _____ Wash feet daily.

   _____ Use lotion daily.

15. Diabetic ketoacidosis (DKA) is a medical emergency caused by

   _____.

Exercise 2

Virtual Hospital Activity

45 minutes

- Sign in to work at Pacific View Regional Hospital on the Medical-Surgical Floor for Period of Care 1. (*Note:* If you are already in the virtual hospital from a previous exercise, click on **Leave the Floor** and then on **Restart the Program** to get to the sign-in window.)
- From the Patient List, select Harry George (Room 401).
- Click on **Get Report** and read the shift report.
- Click on **Go to Nurses' Station** and then on **Chart**.
- Click on **401** to open Harry George's chart.
- Inside the chart, click on **Emergency Department** and review the information given.

1. What is Harry George's chief complaint upon arrival to the Emergency Department?

2. Upon arrival to the Emergency Department, Harry George's blood glucose level was

   _____.

3. Harry George has:
   a. gestational diabetes.
   b. type 1 diabetes mellitus.
   c. type 2 diabetes mellitus.

4. At 1700 the Emergency Department nurse administered regular insulin 10 units subcutaneously to Harry George. This medicine will begin to work at:
   a. 1715.
   b. 1730.
   c. 1900.
   d. 1930.

5. Peak action of the insulin administered to Harry George will take place between

   _____ and _____.

6. The insulin administered to Harry George will demonstrate effectiveness until

   _____ to _____.

7. The insulin administered to Harry George is termed:
   a. rapid-acting.
   b. short-acting.
   c. intermediate-acting.
   d. long-acting.

→ • Click on and review the **Laboratory Reports**.

8. Harry George has had an HbA$_{1C}$ test ordered. What information does this test provide? What do the results of Harry George's test indicate about his condition? (*Hint:* Consult your lab reference.)

→ • Click on and review the **Physician's Orders**.

9. The physician has ordered a(n) _____-calorie ADA diet.

10. When planning the diet for Harry George, the nurse knows that what percentage of calories should come from protein?
   a. 10%
   b. 15%-20%
   c. 25%
   d. 30%-35%

11. What schedule has the physician used for the blood glucose checks on Harry George?

12. What impact can illness have on Harry George's diabetes?

13. Insulin dosages are based on the total grams of _____ to be ingested.

→ • Click on **Return to Nurses' Station**.
   • Click on **401** at the bottom of the screen.
   • Click on **Take Vital Signs** and review.
   • Review the Initial Observations.
   • Click on and review the **Clinical Alerts**.
   • Click on **Patient Care** and then on **Physical Assessment**.
   • Complete a head-to-toe assessment by clicking on the body system categories (yellow buttons) and subsystem categories (green buttons).

14. Harry George's fasting blood glucose at 0730 was _____.

→ • Click on **MAR**; then click on tab **401**.
   • Review the medications ordered.

15. What oral medication has been ordered to manage Harry George's diabetes?

16. The medication you identified in the preceding question belongs to which classification?
    (*Hint:* Consult the Drug Guide.)
    a. Sulfonylureas
    b. Meglitinides
    c. D-phenylalanines
    d. Biguanides
    e. Alpha-glucosidase inhibitors
    f. Thiazolidinediones

17. This medication works by:
    a. promoting insulin secretion by the pancreas.
    b. decreasing glucose production by the liver and increasing glucose uptake by muscle.
    c. inhibiting carbohydrate digestion and absorption.
    d. decreasing insulin resistance.

Care of Patients with Substance Abuse Disorders

Reading Assignment: Care of Patients with Substance Abuse Disorders (Chapter 47)

Patient: Harry George, Medical-Surgical Floor, Room 401

Objectives:

1. Explain the differences among abuse, dependence, and tolerance.
2. Review the physical, behavioral, and psychologic manifestations of substance use.
3. Identify defense mechanisms used by individuals experiencing substance abuse.
4. Discuss symptoms and complications of withdrawal from alcohol.

Exercise 1

Writing Activity

 30 minutes

1. _____ refers to the excessive use of drugs or alcohol.

2. Psychoactive substances are any mind-altering agents capable of changing a person's

   _____, _____,

   _____, _____, or

   _____.

3. _____ The terms *addiction* and *tolerance* are interchangeable. (True/False)

4. During a discussion of a patient's history of substance abuse, the patient reports that he drinks to help himself relax. Which of the following defense mechanisms is the patient demonstrating?
   a. Denial
   b. Rationalization
   c. Enabling
   d. Regression

5. Match each of the following defense mechanisms with its correct description.

Defense Mechanism	Description
_____ Denial	a. Rechanneling an impulse into a more socially desirable acceptable activity
_____ Displacement	
_____ Identification	b. Discharging intense feelings for one person onto another object or person considered to be less threatening
_____ Intellectualization	c. Excessive reasoning and logic to counter emotional distress
_____ Splitting	
_____ Sublimation	d. Ignoring reality
	e. Modeling behavior after someone else
	f. Viewing people or situations as all good or all bad

6. When caring for a patient suspected of abusing marijuana, the nurse can expect to observe which of the following symptoms? Select all that apply.

_____ Euphoria

_____ Reduced inhibitions

_____ Drowsiness

_____ Reduced respiratory rate

_____ Ataxia

_____ Increased appetite

7. A patient is beginning to withdraw from narcotic analgesics. What manifestations may be anticipated?
   a. Watery eyes
   b. Increased alertness
   c. Long periods of sleep
   d. Illusions

8. A patient informs the nurse that he takes "crystal" on occasion. The nurse knows that this drug is also referred to by which of the following names? Select all that apply.

_____ Vicodin

_____ Downers

_____ Speed

_____ Methamphetamine

_____ Crank

9. A patient begins to experience feelings typically associated with drug use despite being

   drug-free. The patient may be experiencing a _____.

10. An assessment used to review for alcohol abuse is the _____.

11. _____ Withdrawal from an opiate may be life-threatening. (True/False)

12. _____ Acupuncture may be used to assist patients in alcohol and drug recovery
    programs. (True/False)

13. _____ Smoking is increasing in the United States. (True/False)

Exercise 2

Virtual Hospital Activity

30 minutes

- Sign in to work at Pacific View Regional Hospital on the Medical-Surgical Floor for Period
  of Care 2. (*Note:* If you are already in the Virtual Hospital from a previous exercise, click on
  Leave the Floor and then on **Restart the Program** to get to the sign-in window.)
- From the Patient List, select Harry George, Room 401.
- Click on **Get Report** and read the shift report.
- Click on **Go to Nurses' Station**.
- Click on **Chart** and then on **401**.
- Click on and review the **Nursing Admission** and **History and Physical**.

1. What is Harry George's diagnosis?

2. Alcohol use has been a problem for Harry George for _____ years.

3. In addition to alcohol use, what substances does Harry George use on a regular basis?

4. Harry has smoked _____ packs of cigarettes per day for _____ years.

5. Name three psychosocial issues that will have an impact on Harry George's potential for recovery from alcohol abuse.

6. When did Harry George last have alcohol?

7. The signs of alcohol withdrawal will begin within _____ to _____ hours after the last drink of alcohol.

→ • Click on and review the **Physician's Orders**.

8. What medication has been ordered to manage Harry George's agitation?
   a. Gentamicin
   b. Folic acid
   c. Cefotaxime
   d. Chlordiazepoxide hydrochloride

9. _____ has been ordered to prevent seizures during Harry George's period of withdrawal from alcohol.

10. Thiamine has been prescribed by the physician. What is the best rationale for its use?
    a. Suppress CNS activity
    b. Correct nutritional deficiencies
    c. Reduce ataxia
    d. Reduce the incidence of confusion

→ • Click on **Return to Nurses' Station**.
   • Click on **401** at the bottom of the screen.
   • Review the Initial Observations.
   • Click on **Clinical Alerts** and review.
   • Click on **Patient Care** and then on **Physical Assessment**.
   • Complete a full body assessment by clicking on the body system categories (yellow buttons) and subcategories (green buttons).

11. Name three behaviors being exhibited by Harry George that are consistent with alcohol withdrawal.

12. When preparing the plan of care for Harry George, the nurse must remember that alcohol withdrawal symptoms may last for how long?
    a. Up to 24 hours
    b. 1-2 days
    c. 3-5 days
    d. 5-7 days

13. _____ Harry George's blood pressure is likely reduced in response to his alcohol withdrawal. (True/False)

14. Identify at least five complementary and alternative therapies that may be employed to manage Harry George's pain.

15. _____ Harry George is a candidate for Antabuse at this time. (True/False)

LESSON 14

Mental Health Care: Patients with Anxiety and Thought Disorders

Reading Assignment: Care of Patients with Anxiety, Mood, and Eating Disorders
(Chapter 46)
Care of Patients with Thought and Personality Disorders
(Chapter 49)

Patient: Jacquline Catanazaro, Medical-Surgical Floor, Room 402

Objectives:

1. Identify descriptions of common anxiety disorders.
2. List factors that may influence mental health.
3. Review the differing types of schizophrenia.
4. Identify behaviors that may manifest in a patient experiencing a thought or personality disorder.

Exercise 1

Writing Activity

30 minutes

1. Match each of the following anxiety disorders with its correct description.

Anxiety Disorder	Description
_____ Generalized anxiety disorder (GAD)	a. Recurrent or intrusive thoughts that cause anxiety
_____ Phobic disorder	b. Persistent, unrealistic, or excessive worry about two or more life circumstances
_____ Obsessive-compulsive disorder (OCD)	c. Intense horror, with recurrent symptoms of anxiety and nightmares, or flashbacks after experiencing an extreme life-threatening event
_____ Posttraumatic stress disorder (PTSD)	d. Excessive fear of a situation or object

2. The _____
   provides a set of diagnostic criteria (specific behaviors) and a specific time frame for each
   mental health disorder.

3. A physician has ordered lorazepam (Ativan) for a patient experiencing anxiety. Which of
   the following factors should the nurse understand about this medication?
   a. It has a depressant action on the central nervous system (CNS).
   b. It is always ordered as a scheduled medication, never prn.
   c. It is associated with tolerance.
   d. It is associated with dependence.

4. A patient demonstrates unstable and frequently changing behaviors. The term to describe

   this patient's actions is _____.

5. A patient with _____ exhibits episodes of extreme
   sadness, hopelessness, and helplessness interspersed with periods of extreme elation and
   hyperactivity.

6. Major depressive disorder is suspected in a patient. Which of the following criteria may be
   used to confirm the diagnosis? Select all that apply.

   _____ An overwhelming feeling of sadness

   _____ Ability to feel pleasure and interest in activities only for short periods of time

   _____ Weight loss not attributed to any form of dieting

   _____ Difficulty making decisions

   _____ Rapid thought processes

   _____ Difficulty concentrating

7. _____ A patient taking monoamine oxidase inhibitors (MAOIs) should avoid eating
             salty foods. (True/False)

8. _____ Combining MAOIs or selective serotonin reuptake inhibitors (SSRIs) with
             St. John's wort can cause adverse drug-herb reactions. (True/False)

9. The most common thought disorder is _____.

10. A patient is experiencing negative symptoms. Which of the following may be included in
    this description? Select all that apply.

    _____ Apathy

    _____ Fatigue

    _____ Limited motivation

    _____ Lack of motivation

    _____ Inability to experience pleasure

11. A patient with schizophrenia is sitting in stupor and is rigid with exopraxia and echolalia. What type of schizophrenia is the patient exhibiting?
    a. Paranoid
    b. Catatonic
    c. Disorganized
    d. Undifferentiated
    e. Residual

12. List at least six factors that affect coping with illness.

13. After a stressful day at work, an individual comes home and harshly disciplines her children. Which of the following defense mechanisms is the person demonstrating?
    a. Identification
    b. Isolation
    c. Displacement
    d. Projection

14. The external presentation of a person's feeling state and emotional responsiveness is

    referred to as the _____.

15. _____ A patient is seen repeatedly washing her hands. This action is referred to as an obsession. (True/False)

16. _____ St. John's wort is commonly used to relieve depression. (True/False)

Exercise 2

 Virtual Hospital Activity

30 minutes

- Sign in to work at Pacific View Regional Hospital on the Medical-Surgical Floor for Period of Care 1. (*Note:* If you are already in the Virtual Hospital form a previous exercise, click on **Leave the Floor** and then on **Restart the Program** to get to the sign-in window.)
- From the Patient List, select Jacquline Catanazaro (Room 402).
- Click on **Get Report** and read the shift report.

1. Describe the psychologic behaviors documented in the two shift reports.

2. _____ Anxiety could increase Jacquline Catanazaro's respiratory distress. (True/False)

- Click on **Go to Nurses' Station**.
- Click on **Chart** and then on **402**.
- Click on **Emergency Department** and review.

3. According to the records, Jacquline Catanazaro has not taken her prescribed schizophrenia

   medications for _____ days or her asthma medications for _____ days.

- Click on **Consultations** and review.

4. What consultations have been ordered by the physician to assist Jacquline Catanazaro?

5. When was Jacquline Catanazaro diagnosed with schizophrenia?

6. What manifestations are associated with psychotic symptoms?

7. Discuss the plan outlined in Jacquline Catanazaro's Psychiatric Consult. (*Hint:* Return to the **Consultations** tab in her chart if necessary.)

➡ • Click on and review the **Nursing Admission**.

8. _____ Jacquline Catanazaro has a family history of mental illness. (True/False)

9. To what does Jacquline Catanazaro attribute her lack of compliance with her prescribed medications?
   a. Financial concerns
   b. Belief that the medications are dangerous for her
   c. Concerns about the side effects of the medications on her weight
   d. Inability to remember to take medications

10. From whom does Jacquline Catanazaro get most of her social support?
    a. Her estranged husband
    b. Her sister
    c. Her adult children
    d. Her parents

11. Discuss Jacquline Catanazaro's use of alcohol and drugs.

12. How has the exacerbation of Jacquline Catanazaro's illness affected her sleep patterns?

13. Evaluate Jacquline Catanazaro's participation in her care at the time of her illness.
    a. Active participant
    b. Moderately active participant
    c. Passive in participation with her care

14. What are Jacquline Catanazaro's primary concerns about being admitted to the hospital?
    a. Fear of losing independence
    b. Concern about financial responsibility for hospital bills
    c. Fear of being poisoned by the medications prescribed
    d. Inability to be discharged in a timely manner

→ • Click on **Return to Nurses' Station**.
   • Click on **MAR** and select tab **402**.

15. _____ has been prescribed to manage Jacquline Catanazaro's schizophrenia.

16. When the nurse administers the medication you identified in the preceding question, what nursing implication should be observed?
    a. Administer on an empty stomach
    b. Administer with meals
    c. Administer at bedtime
    d. Administer with milk

LESSON 15

Mental Health Care: Patients with Cognitive Disorders

Reading Assignment: Care of Patients with Cognitive Disorders (Chapter 48)

Patient: William Jefferson, Skilled Nursing Floor, Room 501

Objectives:

1. Identify nursing interventions that can be used to promote rapport when caring for the patient experiencing confusion.
2. List medications used to manage patients experiencing altered mental states.
3. Review potential causes of altered mental states.

Exercise 1

 Writing Activity

 30 minutes

1. How do delirium and dementia differ?

2. _____ Alzheimer's disease is a type of dementia. (True/False)

3. Which of the following may be causes of delirium? Select all that apply.

_____ Cerebrovascular accident

_____ Drug overdose

_____ Systemic infections

_____ Malnutrition

_____ Elevated blood glucose levels

_____ Fluid and electrolyte imbalances

4. Listed below are terms associated with alterations in cognition. Match each term with its correct description.

Term	Description
_____ Illusion	a. Seeing or hearing things that are not present
_____ Hallucination	b. Belief in a false idea
_____ Delusion	c. A misinterpretation of reality

5. Which of the following factors put older adults at an increased risk for substance-induced delirium? Select all that apply.

_____ Reduced kidney function

_____ Venous stasis

_____ Increased incidence of cardiovascular disease

_____ Reduced liver function

_____ Increased metabolism

6. _____ refers to making up experiences to fill conversation gaps.

7. Any type of dementia caused by vessel disease is known as

_____.

8. Discuss the relationship between the terms *mood* and *affect*.

9. A nurse is preparing a plan of care for a patient with dementia. What is the minimum amount of sleep the patient needs in a 24-hour period?
   a. 4 hours
   b. 6 hours
   c. 8 hours
   d. 9 hours

10. _____ Mirrors can stimulate communication with patients with dementia. (True/False)

11. When caring for a patient who needs restraints, the nurse knows that the restrained area

    must be assessed at least every _____ hours.

12. Which of the following may be useful and therapeutic when caring for a patient with dementia? Select all that apply.

    _____ Elderspeak

    _____ Massage

    _____ Aromatherapy

    _____ Acupuncture

    _____ Restraints

Exercise 2

 Virtual Hospital Activity

 30 minutes

- Sign in to work at Pacific View Regional Hospital on the Skilled Nursing Floor for Period of Care 1. (*Note:* If you are already in the virtual hospital from a previous exercise, click on **Leave the Floor** and then on **Restart the Program** to get to the sign-in window.)
- From the Patient List, select William Jefferson (Room 501).
- Click on **Get Report** and read the shift report.
- Click on **Go to Nurses' Station**.
- Click on **Chart** and then on **501**.
- Click on and review the **Physician's Orders**, **Physician's Notes**, **Nursing Admission**, and **History and Physical**.

1. What is William Jefferson's chief complaint?

2. List at least three of William Jefferson's other health concerns.

3. _____ African Americans have a greater risk for the development of Alzheimer's disease than do whites. (True/False)

4. _____ Alzheimer's disease is fatal. (True/False)

5. Which of the following characteristics pertaining to William Jefferson are considered risk factors that may increase his likelihood for the development of vascular dementia? Select all that apply.

_____ Hyperlipidemia

_____ Hypertension

_____ Diabetes mellitus

_____ History of social drinking

_____ History of tobacco use

6. Who are the primary care providers for William Jefferson?

7. You are preparing to assess the patient for the presence and degree of delirium or dementia. What parameters should be included in your assessment?

8. What psychosocial issues could affect the nurse's interaction with William Jefferson? How might these behaviors affect the interaction?

9. Which of the following interventions will assist the nurse in establishing a positive rapport when communicating with William Jefferson? Select all that apply.

_____ Assist the patient to the dining room to promote feelings of socialization.

_____ Face him during the interaction.

_____ Avoid analgesic administration to reduce drowsiness during the interaction.

_____ Provide adequate lighting during the exchange.

_____ Use touch as culturally appropriate.

10. _____ William Jefferson's symptoms can best be described as "sundowning." (True/False)

11. Based on his clinical manifestations, in which stage of Alzheimer's disease does William Jefferson best fit?
   a. Early (mild) stage
   b. Middle (moderate) stage
   c. Middle to late (moderate to severe) stage
   d. Late stage

   • From the chart, click on **Return to Nurses' Station**.
   • Click on **501** at the bottom of the screen.
   • Click on **Patient Care** and then on **Nurse-Client Interactions**.
   • Select and view the video titled **0730: Intervention—Patient Safety**. (*Note:* Check the virtual clock to see whether enough time has elapsed. You can use the fast-forward feature to advance the time by 2-minute intervals if the video is not yet available. Then click again on **Patient Care** and on **Nurse-Client Interactions** to refresh the screen.)

12. During the interaction, what communication techniques are used by the nurse?

   • Click on **MAR** and select tab **501**.
   • Review William Jefferson's ordered medications.

13. Rivastigmine has been ordered to manage William Jefferson's Alzheimer's disease. Which of the following nursing implications are appropriate with this medication?
   a. Administer at bedtime.
   b. Administer prepared dosages within 4 hours.
   c. Mix with milk.
   d. Monitor intake and output.

14. The physician has prescribed _____ mg of rivastigmine BID.

15. The correct dosage of rivastigmine for William Jefferson is:
   a. 45 mL.
   b. 2 mL.
   c. 2.25 mL.
   d. 4.5 mL.

16. When the nurse is administering rivastigmine to William Jefferson, what nursing considerations should be included?

17. Continue to review William Jefferson's ordered medications. Which of the medications will require caution when ordered in conjunction with rivastigmine?
    a. Metformin
    b. Hydrochlorothiazide
    c. Rosiglitazone
    d. Atenolol
    e. Ciprofloxacin
    f. Ibuprofen
    g. Magnesium hydroxide
    h. Lisinopril
    i. Enalapril

18. When administering rivastigmine to William Jefferson, which of the following instructions should be included? Select all that apply.

    _____ Crush the medication to facilitate swallowing.

    _____ Administer medication with meals.

    _____ Report nausea, vomiting, or abdominal pain.

    _____ Assess for urinary retention, which is a serious complication of the medication therapy.

    _____ Administer medication at bedtime.

NOTES:

NOTES:

NOTES:

NOTES:

NOTES:

NOTES:

NOTES: